Know Your Genes

Know Your Genes

Aubrey Milunsky, M.D.

ILLUSTRATED WITH
PHOTOGRAPHS AND DIAGRAMS

Houghton Mifflin Company Boston

Library of Congress Cataloging in Publication Data
Milunsky, Aubrey.
    Know your genes.
    Includes index.
    1. Medical genetics.   I. Title.
RB155.M54   616'.042   77-2274
ISBN 0-395-25374-8

Printed in the United States of America

V 10 9 8 7 6 5 4 3 2

To Babette and Jeff

If, of all words of tongue and pen,
The saddest are, "It might have been,"
More sad are these we daily see:
"It is, but hadn't ought to be."

— FRANCIS BRET HARTE
in "Mrs. Judge Jenkins"

Acknowledgments

THE INFORMATION presented in this book is based upon the research of thousands of people. All the information provided has a scientific basis and a recognized source. I felt, however, that it was inappropriate to list the many hundreds of medical books and journals used. I pay tribute to all these workers whose contributions collectively now provide us with knowledge about genetics that we can apply to our everyday health care.

The sterling work of my secretary, Mrs. Carmela M. Ryan, on yet another book, is again acknowledged with gratitude. In the midst of competing deadlines, she has again efficiently and coolly steered another project to its completion on time.

I am indebted to my research assistant, Ms. Judy Heck, for her untiring efforts. I am in particular appreciative of her resourcefulness.

I am indebted to Dr. L. Atkins for the photographs of the chromosomes.

The editorial assistance of Mrs. Gerta Prosser is gratefully acknowledged. My thanks are especially due to Mr. David Harris and Mr. Austin Olney for their warmth and wise counsel, which simply made the challenge even more fulfilling.

My wife, Babette, provided invaluable assistance and wise counsel throughout this effort. Many of her perspectives and approaches are encompassed within these pages. Her devotion, companionship, and counsel are acknowledged with gratitude.

Preface

"IF ONLY I HAD KNOWN!" is the all too frequent lament that falls on the ears of physicians. It may follow the birth of a child with a serious birth defect, genetic disease, or mental retardation that could have been averted. Or it may refer to personal illness from complications of hereditary disease that could have been avoided or treated.

Recent advances in medicine have now made it possible to prevent tragedies, for example, prior to the birth of a child with an irreparable physical or mental defect. Moreover, it is possible to know, without extensive knowledge of biology or genetics, what your risks are in a given situation, what tests are available, and what options exist. Indeed, I believe *you have a right to know* about your genes, and should have the freedom to exercise your options.

Each of us carries a number of harmful genes and may develop a genetic disorder or transmit one to our children. Every disease is either caused or influenced by genetic mechanisms. Common examples include heart disease, high blood pressure, cancer, diabetes, and allergies. Even longevity is genetically influenced.

Know Your Genes has been written especially for those who have genetic disease, have or have had affected children or relatives, are still to choose a mate, are still to have children, or who care about themselves and their loved ones.

If *Know Your Genes* helps a few families to prevent unnecessary agony, anguish, and suffering, the effort will have been worthwhile. It would be a blessing to be confronted less often by anguished people with their genetic afflictions or those of their children and to find myself thinking sadly, "It is, but hadn't ought to be!"

AUBREY MILUNSKY

Boston, January 1977

Contents

Chromosomes and Genes

Birth Defects and Genetic Counseling

Will Your Baby Be Normal?

Heredity, Disease, and Aging

Sex, Twins, Ethics, and the Future

Know Your Genes

CHAPTER 1

Why You Should Know

YOU ARE A CARRIER OF FOUR TO EIGHT DIFFERENT HEREDITARY DISEASES! AND SO ARE WE ALL! Since you definitely possess certain harmful genes, you may already have or could develop a hereditary (genetic) disease. Your harmful genes may not, however, have any significant effect on your own health but they make you a carrier capable of transmitting these genes to your children. It is likely that you are unaware of your potential to transmit or even to develop genetic disease, and may not realize the extent of the problem posed by the frequency of genetic disease, birth defects, or mental retardation.

Why the Problem Affects You

For the United States alone, over 20 million people, at least 1 in 10 individuals, has, or will later develop, some disorder that has been inherited. This does not have to be. That is why I have written this book: to elucidate the many ways in which tragedy can be prevented *in advance,* or treatment initiated *in time.*

In these pages I shall emphasize the distinct hereditary diseases carried by various ethnic or racial groups: Irish, Italians, Greeks, Jews, Orientals, blacks, and whites. There is, for instance, a hereditary disease that affects one white child in about every 2500: cystic fibrosis. Ashkenazic and Sephardic Jews, for example, carry different genetic diseases. There are also many, many inherited diseases that have nothing to do with racial origins.

Certainly it should not have to take the birth of a child with an irreparable defect to alert you to the possibility of just such an event. Science now provides many tests that help us to prevent or, at least, successfully treat the hereditary disorder obvious at birth or that crops up later in life.

There is no family, and no person planning to have a child, who can morally ignore the new genetic discoveries and techniques of preventing genetic disease. Your health and welfare and that of your (future) children are at stake here. We all have a right and, indeed, an obligation to know about our particular genes and to consider the options available that enable us to have healthy children. We should also all have the *freedom* to exercise these options as we wish and as rationally as we are able.

Over two thousand genetic diseases have been identified. It is therefore not surprising that they amount to 25 to 30 percent of admissions into the major children's hospitals in the United States and Canada. This large proportion is, of course, due partly to the waning of serious infectious diseases over the last few decades, as well as to improved early recognition of these disorders, and an increased lifespan for some of them.

About 3 to 4 in every 100 babies are born with major birth defects. There are, moreover, over 6 million persons in the United States who, for either hereditary or congenital reasons, are mentally retarded.

This is frightening, you may say. Enough, you say, we have heard all that before! But many types of genetic diseases are barely known about and hardly ever mentioned.

Various Types of Hereditary Disorders

Troubles that "run in the family" are apt to be glossed over so that people often do not really know much about what they may have inherited. Often we don't want to know; but that is an indulgence for which we may pay dearly. Each of us may inherit a disease directly, from one parent who is affected, say, by Huntington's chorea, a progressive deterioration of brain tissue causing dementia and purposeless muscle movements and speech defects. A disease such as cystic fibrosis, causing chronic lung infection and malabsorption of food, is transmitted by two parents who are completely healthy and may themselves never have heard about the disease, though they carry it in their genes. Tay-Sachs disease, a disorder that causes brain destruction, blindness, and eventually death and found almost exclusively in the Jewish Ashkenazic ethnic group, is also caused by genes transmitted from both parents. Similarly, blacks transmit the genes causing sickle cell anemia to their progeny.

Hemophilia, a bleeding disease due to a missing blood-clotting factor, is transmitted only by females but occurs almost always in males. It is not special to any race (though it has been associated with the highly inbred European royalty). Open spine defects, more common among people with Irish ancestry, may also occur in all races. High blood pressure, coronary heart disease, cancer, diabetes, mental retardation, schizophrenia, and skin disorders like eczema may also be inherited by anyone, anywhere.

Willy-nilly, we are involved in our genes. In a way, we *are* our genes.

An Inherited Predisposition

You may believe you are in perfectly good health, and it is to be hoped that you are. Many of us, however, through our genetic endowment — our genes — are predisposed to react in a specific way, a possibly fatal way, to certain environmental agents. For example, you may appear to be perfectly healthy, but have nevertheless a particular enzyme (a substance involved in the normal making and breaking down of body chemicals) missing from your red blood cells. When exposed to some drugs (even aspirin or sulfa drugs) a severe reaction may occur or a hemolytic anemia may develop. Greeks, Italians, Orientals, blacks, and other groups may be especially prone to such reactions because of this enzyme (glucose-6-phosphate dehydrogenase) deficiency. Fatal reactions to penicillin are probably also genetically determined, but in a different way. Another alarming phenomenon is the fatal reaction to general anesthesia of apparently healthy individuals who may have a particular hereditary muscle disease not ordinarily evident. During or after their operation under general anesthesia, they may suddenly develop an extraordinarily high fever (such as a body temperature of 108° F) and die from a complication unrelated to the disorder for which they had been operated upon.

Of particular special interest is the recent recognition that certain persons possess a particular enzyme whose activation may lead to the development of cancer. For example, a person may activate this enzyme by heavy smoking, thereby leading to the occurrence of lung cancer. It might also explain why certain people who have smoked heavily throughout their lives have never developed lung cancer; they simply do not possess or do not activate this particular enzyme.

Why Know Now?

Knowledge about many hereditary diseases has been available for years, so why the urgency to press you now about these matters? Until relatively recently there were more pressing problems that took priority over genetic diseases, and this is still the case in many underdeveloped parts of the world. Malnutrition and infectious disorders are the primary problems that require attention before a society can turn to more sophisticated considerations, including the management and prevention of hereditary diseases.

But today it is possible to *prevent* many hereditary disorders, and it is urgent that you should *know about your risks and options*. These options include choosing your mate; having tests to determine if you are a carrier of a genetic disorder; having prenatal testing in pregnancy to diagnose particular fetal defects; or simply through genetic counseling, discovering what risks you have yourself, and what risks there are for having defective offspring. It is crucial to keep things in *perspective*, however, since about 96 percent of all children are born free of genetic diseases, major birth defects, or mental retardation.

A Right to Know

You have a right to know if your risks for having defective children are higher than normal, if you are a carrier of specific hereditary disorders, and what tests or other options are available to you. True, you also owe it to yourself and your future children to know your family history, to seek consultations from specialists, and to take advantage of the recent advances in medical technology that allow for the prevention of genetic diseases.

None of us would like to discover that we have a hereditary disease, or that one of our children is affected, especially when that particular disorder was preventable. Certainly there are those individuals who, because of their religious beliefs or other reasons, while not wishing to have children affected by hereditary disease, choose not to interfere with what they regard as their destiny, or God's will, and would not consider abortion of a defective fetus. This is their free prerogative, and such action and belief must be safeguarded. For those, however, who select the option to prevent serious or fatal genetic disease, their rights too must be protected.

On the other hand, the responsibility to one's mate prior to marriage is self-evident. Surely children have the right to be born free of birth defects and serious or fatal hereditary disease? Indeed the Supreme Court of Rhode Island has spoken explicitly to this point:

> Justice requires that the principle be recognized that a child has a legal right to begin life with a sound mind and body.

In order to ensure this right, all prospective parents have to act in a responsible way by determining if they are indeed carriers or personally at risk for having a genetic disease.

Society, too, has a stake in your actions and how you perceive your responsibilities. If you choose simply to have children with serious hereditary disease, who, for example, also have mental retardation, the state will inevitably end up being responsible — sooner or later, and in one way or another —

for the care of your affected offspring. We will explore the morality and ethics of some of these problems and approaches later (see Chapters 22 and 23).

Minor and Major Birth Defects

There is of course great variation in the severity of birth defects. Minor ones are very common; some researchers suggest they occur in 6 to 14 percent of live births. You may well have some yourself. Do you, for example, have a single crease across your palm? While this so-called simian crease occurs very frequently in Down's syndrome (mongolism), a single transverse palmar crease is also found on one or both hands in about 1 percent of healthy, normal newborns, who, strangely enough, are more commonly male first-borns. Are your second and third toes webbed or bunched? Perhaps one of your parents has a similar minor defect. Are your fifth fingers slightly incurved? Do you have flat feet? How many birthmarks? Do your ears have an unusual shape? Is your palate high-arched? All of these minor birth defects occurring in an isolated fashion usually have no significant meaning. On occasion, however, even minor defects may signal the presence of an associated major birth defect. For example, if one of your ears was shaped very differently than the other, the kidney on the side of the abnormally shaped ear may also be abnormal, and that could be very important to your health!

In contrast, major birth defects are of course more serious, by being life-threatening or disfiguring. Heart defects, very small heads (microcephaly), mental retardation, blindness, deafness, dwarfism, and many others are in this category.

Inherited or Acquired Birth Defects

Both major and minor defects may occur "out of the blue" without any cause ever being determined. Certain medications taken during pregnancy (e.g., thalidomide) or a suspected viral illness in early pregnancy (e.g., German measles) may be considered in trying to evaluate the cause. The condition, of course, may be hereditary. Not infrequently problems are encountered in trying to differentiate an acquired (e.g., caused by a drug or virus) defect from one that has genetic origins, even though no previous cases have occurred in the entire family. Individuals with hereditary diseases may be born with gross disfiguring abnormalities; or show no evidence of the particular disease for months or even decades (e.g., Tay-Sachs disease, Huntington's chorea); or die within hours or days from irremediable biochemical faults in metabolism; irreparable mental retardation may become apparent only many months after birth.

An infant born with an abnormality may merely have suffered from some trauma in early intrauterine life. Babies who suffer from lack of oxygen or are brain damaged in some way during the hours before, during, or immediately after delivery may later be found to have cerebral palsy, mental retardation, or epilepsy. These very sad instances of damage occur in what up to that moment has usually been a *normal* fetus. These *acquired* conditions causing brain injury will not specifically be discussed in this book, the main thrust of which is a consideration of hereditary disease and defective development.

Options

In the past the only possible approach by the physician — because so little was known — was simply to await the birth of a child with a serious genetic disease. Only at that point was it possible to counsel the parents about their exact risk of recurrence in subsequent pregnancies, for example, 25 percent for recessive diseases (see Chapter 5). The newest advances in many hereditary disorders make it possible to diagnose genetic disease actually in the fetus. It is therefore critically important that families with serious problems of this kind remain in contact with major medical centers providing sophisticated genetic counseling, in order to benefit from continuing new discoveries.

The following is a good case in point:

Mary and Joe were twenty-three and twenty-four years old respectively when they married. Both were perfectly well themselves. Mary's brother, however, had died at the age of fifteen from muscular dystrophy. At the time of her brother's death, the parents were told that Mary was indeed a possible carrier of muscular dystrophy and was therefore at risk for having male offspring with this disease. No effort was made to actually determine if she was a carrier, and as the years rolled by and Mary's marriage approached, no one suggested genetic counseling again. The very first pregnancy yielded a beautiful boy who appeared entirely normal. However, when his son was three and a half years old, Joe noticed that he had difficulty climbing the stairs and even getting up from a sitting position on the floor. The diagnosis of muscular dystrophy was made in the same week that Mary's second pregnancy was confirmed.

The attending general practitioner counseled the parents that Mary indeed was a carrier (confirmed by a blood test) and that in the future she would have a 50 percent risk that any male offspring would be affected by muscular dystrophy. The physician advised, however, that in the preceding year it had become possible to predict fetal sex early enough in pregnancy to offer the parents an elective abortion if a male fetus was indeed found. Mary and Joe opted for the amniocentesis test that showed that the fetus was a male, and they elected to terminate the pregnancy. Using prenatal diagnosis studies, they subsequently had two normal girls.

There is much that is new in clinical genetics today, and it takes major efforts by practicing physicians to keep up with the latest recommendations stemming from advances in genetics as well as in all other fields. It is not, however, possible for any physician to know the answers about all the various complex problems in medicine, though he or she can reasonably be expected to seek and to find expert consultation for his or her patient. This applies equally well to medical genetics. Should you at any time feel that you would be happier with another opinion, then it would be entirely reasonable to seek one in a major medical school/hospital center. All physicians should be sufficiently sensitive and secure to offer the very anxious or extremely concerned person an opportunity for a second opinion. Sadly, this is not always true.

Paradoxically, the patient can play an important part by bringing to the attention of a physician a recent advance in medicine culled from the latest weekly magazine, or learned from Know Your Genes. The National Foundation–March of Dimes has done more about care, prevention, and education concerning birth defects than any other charitable group. The National Genetics Foundation, the Hemophilia Foundation, the National Cystic Fibrosis Foundation, the Muscular Dystrophy Association, the Tay-Sachs Foundation, the Committee to Combat Huntington's Chorea, the Sickle Cell Anemia Foundation, and many others have played critical roles in making people aware of the need for genetic counseling.

Having a Defective Child

After the initial shock of learning that the child has a major birth defect or is likely to be severely mentally retarded, a complex set of reactions and adaptive mechanisms generally appears. Depression and feelings of guilt are natural, despite the fact that in the majority of cases no culpability can be ascribed to either parent. On occasion, either the mother or the father or both may refuse to accept the likelihood that their child will be severely retarded. Indeed, their defensive rejection of the probable reality may be so strong as to block reception of any genetic counseling that is provided soon after the birth of the affected child. The result is that even in situations where the risk of having a similarly affected infant is high, another pregnancy is apt to follow rapidly.

Bitterness is common and is occasionally accompanied by envy of close relatives who have normal children. One parent may indulge in self-pity or seek solace in alcohol. Initial anger with the physicians for not having prevented their tragedy often gives rise to a sense of increasing frustration over the inadequacy of care or the lack of a specific diagnosis, treatment, or cure.

The presence of a child with serious birth defects in the home becomes a chronic emotional and physical drain on the parents, leading often to a severe state of exhaustion affecting all avenues of their life. Economic hardship may follow and almost invariably increases marital conflict. The sex life of the couple becomes a major casualty and these problems further feed the fires of anger and frustration. Separation and divorce are only too well known in families where such tragedies have occurred. The enormous drain on the energies of the parents frequently leads to a relative neglect of the unaffected children. Generally speaking, it is simply not possible for parents in this situation to have sufficient energy and time left over to attend to their normal children as they would otherwise have done. As a consequence of this neglect, which is often not recognized, emotional, behavioral, and psychological problems develop in the normal siblings.

These major difficulties can become chronic and provide lifetime complications of one sort or another for all members of the household, though not every family having such a child is as devastated as described. Those sufficiently wealthy to employ full-time help are often the most vocal about how families can and should cope with these tragedies. Try as they might, middle- and lower-income parents often find it impossible to do their best for both the affected child and their other children. It is a very rare family that "benefits" from such catastrophes. True, the qualities of compassion, patience, and love can be brought out by caring for the abnormal child or adult, a healthy adaptation, but unfortunately unusual in most families. All things considered, it is a heavy burden, and feelings of anger, guilt, and frustration are especially bitter when parents realize *too late* that the tragedy could have been prevented.

Science has now made us *responsible* through knowledge and has provided the means to take the fear out of old superstitions and aversions.

I have often witnessed the deep despair of a mother and father when they are told that their tragedy was not inevitable; for, all the time, deep inside, they really did know it, but . . .

All of us have a tendency to postpone action on a health problem until it becomes urgent, and often it is too late. This book is sending you a personal message about a slightly different, equally real, and even more compelling urgency. In the words of Robert Louis Stevenson:

> Let me do it now
> Let me not defer it nor neglect it
> For I shall not pass this way again.

CHAPTER 2

Chromosomes

"BUT WHY US? What are chromosomes? Why does our baby have an extra one? Does it come from either of us? Can it happen again?"

Distraught and bewildered young parents in my consulting room for the first time, still caught in the dismal fog of disbelief and unreality caused by my diagnosis, invariably ask me such questions as soon as they are able to speak at all.

Time and again couples have confided that they have no idea what chromosomes are, their difference from genes, or even the difference between congenital and hereditary defects.

I try to answer as clearly as possible, while assuring them that they need no prior knowledge of biology to understand. The explanation is made simply with the help of a few illustrations and photographs. We begin with the cell.

Cells

Our bodies are made up of billions of cells, many of which have very special functions: brain cells for memory and intelligence, heart cells for rhythmic contraction, intestinal cells for making mucus, and so on. The cells of our bodies live for variable periods of time, depending upon their organs of origin. While we cannot grow new brain cells (in fact we steadily lose brain cells as we get older), the cells lining our intestines are lost and replaced by new ones every 24 hours or so. It has been estimated that about 50 million cells in our bodies die every second and are rapidly replaced by about the same number. Sperm cells in the testes may live only a few months, while ova (eggs) in the ovaries may live longer than 50 years. The implication for birth defects is therefore that a woman's ova are exposed to environmental influences, such as x-rays and drugs, all through her childhood and childbearing life.

Despite their specialized functions, all cells have similar basic component parts. The center of operations within each cell is tiny and is called the nucleus. It controls not only the functions of that cell, but also contains the messages or blueprints inherited from our parents that determine what the cell will actually do, and what characteristics will be passed along to each of our children. Each cell nucleus contains tiny threads of chemical compounds called chromosomes, the most important component of which is DNA (deoxyribonucleic acid).

Normal Chromosomes

It was known almost a century ago that when a special dye was added to a cell at a critical point in its formation, these threadlike structures of protein would take up the dye and stain, becoming easier to see. They were therefore called chromosomes, from the Greek words "chroma" meaning color and "soma" for body. Late in the nineteenth century the chromosomes were already considered to be the likely carriers of hereditary factors.

All the necessary information required to direct the formation and function of a human being — or of any other living thing from bacteria, to plants, to elephants — is contained by these complex thin threads. The chromosomes are, in turn, composed of genes, which are the units of heredity. Single genes are so small that they remain invisible even when looked at by the most modern instruments, including the electron microscope.

We receive half our chromosome complement from our mother and half from our father. The genes constituting the chromosomes are therefore equally contributed to us by each parent. In turn, we will pass along half our chromosomes and genes to each of our own children. A look at what normally happens to chromosomes as they pass from parent to child helps us understand what can happen to chromosomes when things go wrong.

Number, Size, and Sex

The number of chromosomes and their structure vary greatly among living organisms, ranging from 4 to 500 in each cell. Chimpanzees and gorillas have 48 chromosomes per cell. In 1956, humans were shown to have 46 chromosomes in every cell (except sperm and ova, which have 23 each) and not 48 as was previously thought. The chromosomes in a cell can be viewed through the microscope and photographed and appear as shown in Figure 1. Each chromosome in the photograph can be cut out, pasted on cardboard and arranged in order — the largest being first, as shown in Figure 2. There are 22 pairs (a total of 44), which are numbered as shown. One chromosome of each pair is from the father, and the other is from the mother.

The remaining two chromosomes in every cell are called sex chromosomes, since they carry the message that determines which sex the individual will be. Note that the two sex chromosomes are arranged separately in the paste-out (Figure 2). Each parent passes along one sex chromosome to his or her offspring. The two sex chromosomes in females are denoted as XX and in males as XY. When the female contributes a single X, and the male also contributes an X, then the offspring will be a girl (XX). If the male passes along a Y chromosome to combine with the female chromosome, then the newborn child will be a male (XY). The presence of the Y chromosome always dictates that the offspring will be male (even in abnormal states where there are two or even more X chromosomes together with the Y chromosome).

Each chromosome can be distinguished from another even more accurately than by size alone. Using new staining techniques, it is possible to distinguish horizontal bands on every chromosome (Figure 3). Indeed it seems likely that, as with our fingerprints, the banding pattern along each chromosome is unique for each individual person. These new techniques represent important advances because they make it possible to

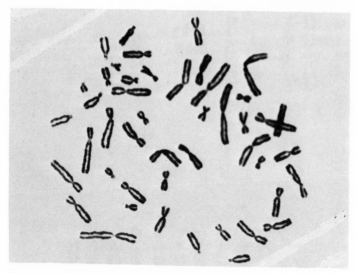

Figure 1   Chromosomes within a cell as seen through the microscope.

detect extremely small defects that could otherwise be missed by the routinely used techniques.

Sperm and Eggs

In the formation of both the sperm and the ovum or egg the usual 46 chromosomes per cell are reduced to half that number: 23 chromosomes. When they fuse at fertilization, they form one cell that again contains 46 chromosomes. How did the sperm and egg form with only 23 chromosomes each? And once fertilization occurred, how did the chromosomes divide as we grow from a single cell into a whole person? The sequence of events is best followed by observing Figure 4 carefully as we go along. Let us start with one cell nucleus in the testis. The same process happens in the ovary. To make it easier, we will follow only one of the 23 pairs of chromosomes in that cell nucleus. The same process, called meiosis, occurs for each of the 23 chromosome pairs in every cell from which sperm or eggs originate.

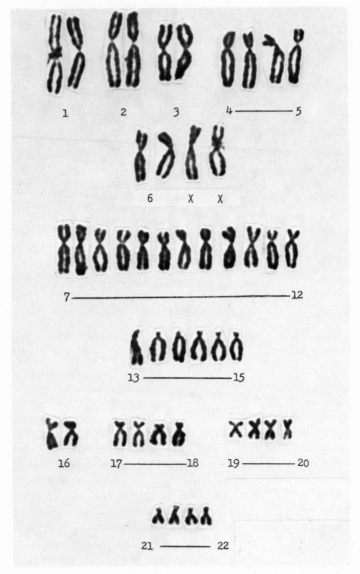

Figure 2   Normal human chromosomes in one cell arranged in descending order of size.

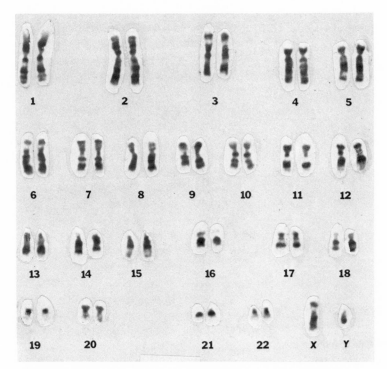

Figure 3 Normal human chromosomes from one cell arranged in descending order of size and stained to demonstrate cross-striations (bands).

Step 1: Shows one cell with a pair of chromosomes.

Step 2: The chromosomes split longitudinally and begin to pair off.

Step 3: The cell nucleus begins to divide.

Step 4: The cell nucleus (and the cell that it occupies) has divided into two new nuclei, each containing a pair of chromosomes.

Step 5: The two chromosomes in each new nucleus now begin to move apart as the cell and its nucleus divide.

Step 6: A new cell and nucleus are formed, each with only one chromosome from the preceding cell. We can

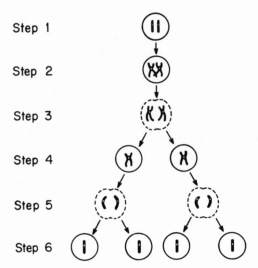

Step 1

Step 2

Step 3

Step 4

Step 5

Step 6

Figure 4   Chromosome division (meiosis) step by step.

see that, from the original cell with a pair of chromosomes, there are four cells each with a single chromosome. These are the sperm cells (or eggs, if in the
ovary) and they obviously contain 23 chromosomes,
which is half of the original number. When a sperm
with 23 chromosomes and an egg with 23 chromosomes meet in fertilization, a single cell is constituted with 46 chromosomes. We have therefore
received half our chromosomes (and therefore genes)
from our father and half from our mother.

Multiplication by Division

We started like this, as a single cell with 46 chromosomes.
Let us follow that single cell (Figure 5) as it divides, a process
called mitosis, and again focus for the sake of simplicity on
only one pair of chromosomes.

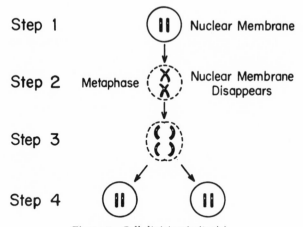

Step 1   Nuclear Membrane

Step 2   Metaphase   Nuclear Membrane Disappears

Step 3

Step 4

Figure 5   Cell division (mitosis).

Step 1:   Shows the single cell with the pair of chromosomes we are following.

Step 2:   The chromosomes split longitudinally, making a total of two pairs.

Step 3:   The chromosome pairs separate; the cell nucleus and the cell itself begin to divide.

Step 4:   One chromosome member of each pair is now found in a new cell. We note that there are two cells from the original single cell. This whole process of cell division continues an infinite number of times to constitute finally all the cells in the human body.

The normal process of cell division may go awry, or chromosomes of the egg or sperm may already be abnormal at the time of fertilization. Either way, the consequences are almost invariably sad. Since chromosomal defects are quite common, we will consider the abnormalities in some detail.

Abnormalities of the Chromosomes

Many specific birth defects or groups of abnormalities or syndromes have been identified with certain abnormalities of individual chromosomes. Chromosomal disorders do occur frequently, about 1 in every 200 live births. In the United States alone, close to 20,000 infants are born each year with chromosomal abnormalities. This figure represents the incidence of abnormalities such as Down's syndrome, which occurs at all ages, as well as abnormalities of the sex chromosomes and those with structural chromosomal defects.

Certainly the chromosomal abnormalities that do occur in the aborted embryos or fetuses are most often extremely serious. Pregnancies with such abnormalities that go to term end with babies affected by gross birth defects such as extremely small heads, deformed brains and faces, cataracts, cleft lips and palates, single nostrils, abnormal ears, poorly formed lower jaws, and heart defects, to name but a few. It should be remembered that virtually every recognizable chromosomal abnormality can be *diagnosed* in the fetus sufficiently early in pregnancy for the parents to consider the option of abortion (see Chapter 15).

Miscarriages

Frequent as chromosomal disorders are in newborns, embryos or fetuses that are spontaneously *miscarried* have a remarkably higher incidence of chromosomal abnormalities. The vast majority (about 45 percent) of chromosomally abnormal fetuses spontaneously miscarried have an extra chromosome in each cell. In contrast, about 20 percent of these miscarriages specifically have a missing X chromosome, a condition called Turner's syndrome, which is discussed in Chapter 3. Since the vast majority of such losses occur in the first three months of pregnancy and so many are defective, many feel and say that miscarriage at this stage is "just as well" or "it is all for the good." Nature, it would seem, acts to rid us of gross malformations.

The Pill

Women taking oral contraceptives have reason to be concerned about the effects on their own bodies. Initially there had also been reason to worry about the effects of the pill on progeny still to be conceived.

During his studies Professor D. H. Carr, in Canada, noted that women who had been on oral contraceptives within a whole six months prior to becoming pregnant had a higher frequency of chromosomal abnormalities in the embryos and produced fetuses that were spontaneously miscarried. He found *no* evidence, however, to suggest that women who had taken oral contraceptives at any other period, including very close to the time they conceived, had given birth to children with a higher frequency of chromosomal abnormalities. Others have confirmed these observations.

New Techniques

The usual techniques used for diagnosing abnormalities of the chromosomes by a microscope do not reveal structural alterations involving less than about one-tenth of a chromosome arm. Use of the new "banding" procedures (see Figure 3) has enhanced our abilities. For example, in one Canadian study routine chromosome-staining techniques were employed in searching for the causes of mental retardation in over 70 children. All the results were initially normal. But application of the new techniques employing "banding" of chromosomes yielded four cases with discernable chromosomal abnormalities — missed by routine approaches. These new techniques are now generally available in most centers.

Too Many or Too Few Chromosomes

Sometimes there are too many chromosomes.

Most commonly such abnormalities arise during the process of cell division. This process is easier to understand if you follow Figure 6. It is the same basic diagram as in Figure 4, steps 1, 2, 3, and 4 being identical. But the crucial differences can be seen in the following steps:

Step 5: The cell nucleus and the cell that it occupies begin to divide into two, but this time the chromosome pair fails to separate.

Step 6: Both remain in one cell, which is now, say, the egg, the other cell ending up with all the other chromosomes but missing this particular one. Most commonly this is the #21 chromosome.

When the egg with the extra chromosome is fertilized by the normal sperm, the resulting single cell has an extra chromosome. The mechanism of chromosome separation could go wrong earlier in the process, for example between steps 3 and 4. The sperm or eggs formed would again end up with either one too many or one too few chromosomes. Any person born with an extra #21 chromosome (Figure 7) in all or many of the cells will have all the features of Down's syndrome (trisomy 21), commonly called mongolism. This, the commonest kind of Down's syndrome, which constitutes about 96 percent of all such offspring, is considered to be nonhereditary. The remaining 4 percent of progeny with Down's syndrome is due to abnormal rearrangements of the chromosomes, which are often hereditary.

The phenomenon of one chromosome sticking with another during cell division, nondisjunction, is not confined to the extra #21 in Down's syndrome, but may occur with #13, #18, or any other chromosome, almost invariably causing serious defects in the child. Of particular interest and importance is that in many of these instances where there is an extra chromosome present, the mother is at least thirty-five years old (see Chapter 15). There is some unknown influence making the extra chromosome stick in these trisomic disorders. Many factors have been suggested as causes, including x-ray exposure (not necessarily during pregnancy!), virus infections, diabetes or thyroid disease of the mother, and even fluoride in drinking water. It has also been repeatedly observed that

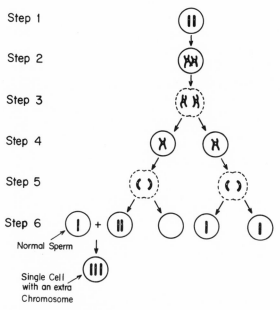

Step 1

Step 2

Step 3

Step 4

Step 5

Step 6

Normal Sperm

Single Cell
with an extra
Chromosome

Figure 6 Abnormal cell division, for example, in the ovary, resulting in one cell with an extra chromosome.

some of the major chromosomal abnormalities, including mongolism, may occur in clusters. A group of affected children may, for example, be born in the same fall or winter. This clue has raised questions about the role of viruses in affecting cell division in the embryo.

The presence of the extra chromosome #21 can be observed under the microscope; it was done for the first time by the French physician Lejeuné and his colleagues in 1959. Such a discovery in a fetus or child means that the parents will ultimately have to face mental retardation, dwarfism, the typical facial features of mongolism, a small head, and other medical, emotional, and social problems. The presence of the extra #13 chromosome usually produces mental retardation, a small head, malformations of the ears and eyes, cleft palate and/or cleft lip, an extra finger on each hand, as well as other abnormalities. The presence of the extra #18 chromosome is

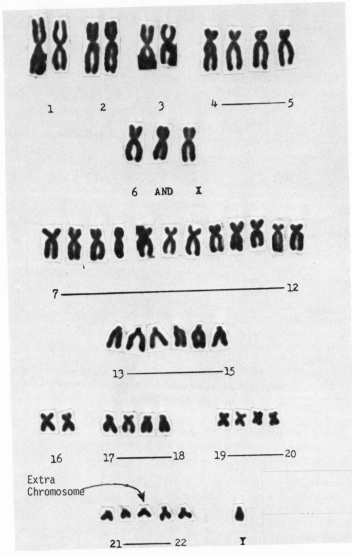

Figure 7 Cell division resulting in an abnormal chromosome number (47) as seen in Down's syndrome. Note: the extra #21 chromosome is typical of this syndrome.

apt to mean mental retardation and defects in ears, eyes, hands, and head.

Very rarely, an infant is born with one too few of the regular, that is, nonsex, chromosomes. In most cases this abnormality is sufficiently serious as to be incompatible with life or, if born alive, the babies have serious birth defects and invariably die soon after birth.

Mixtures of Normal and Abnormal Cells

During the process of cell division there can be a mixture of normal and abnormal cells with two different cell types emerging: one with normal chromosomes and one with an extra chromosome. The resulting individual may finally be made up of a thorough mixture of cells, or certain organs or tissues may be abnormal. For instance, only the brain, the genital organs, the blood, and the skin may have cells with too many chromosomes, with all the other organs having normal cells. Affected individuals are described as having chromosomal *mosaicism.*

If 40 percent of the cells have the normal 46 chromosomes, while 60 percent have the extra #21 chromosome, then the features of mongolism will be present but are likely to be milder, depending upon which organs have normal cells. Generally mosaicism of the regular chromosomes is not common at all (see Chapter 3).

Correct Number of Chromosomes, but Defective Structure

Even when all the chromosomes are present, something may go wrong with one or two of them. These structural abnormalities generally result from breakage. Chromosomes may break spontaneously or result from known (e.g., virus infection) or unrecognized causes operating at the time of conception. The tendency to break can also be transmitted from parent or grandparent to a child. Again these structural chromosomal defects occur fairly commonly: approximately 1 in every 500 live births. A whole variety of changes in chromosomal structure may result from chromosome breakage. For example, two small pieces may break off the end of two different chromosomes and exchange positions. This process is called *translocation* and may occur spontaneously at the time of conception, or be inherited and passed down through the generations. Hereditary Down's syndrome, one type of mongolism, discussed earlier, is the consequence of translocation of certain chromosomes; for example, an exchange between pieces of #14 and #21 chromosomes. When the chromosome pieces change places without any piece or portion being lost in the exchange, the translocation is called a *balanced translocation. Unbalanced translocation* is the term used when some piece or portion is lost, and it is this situation that is associated with serious birth defects and there is a significant likelihood of its recurrence.

There are a fair number of us who, without knowing it, are balanced carriers of various chromosomal abnormalities. Each year in the United States alone about 7000 children are born with balanced or unbalanced chromosomes. Those of us who have a *balanced*-chromosome exchange are at risk of having defective offspring: approximately a 10 to 20 percent risk for prospective mothers and about a 4 percent risk for prospective fathers, depending upon which chromosome is involved. The lower risks for fathers with unbalanced chromosomes suggest that their abnormal sperm don't make it to fertilization. There are some rare situations where the chromosomes are interchanged in such a way as to lead to a child with Down's syndrome *in every pregnancy*: a 100 percent risk!

Recognition of these translocation situations is obviously of critical importance, as shown by the following case (see also Chapter 15):

Jim and Barbara had tried for five years to have a child. Barbara had become pregnant three times during that period, but each time suffered a miscarriage during the second or third month of pregnancy. Because of the recurrent miscarriages, their obstetrician wisely suggested that they both have their chromosomes studied. The results showed that Barbara herself was a balanced translocation carrier for mongolism and it was inferred that at least some of the miscarriages were due to defective embryos. Barbara and Jim were advised that they could still have unaffected children through prenatal genetic studies. This they did in a subsequent pregnancy, the prenatal studies showing a fetus with a balanced translocation and therefore, like Barbara, perfectly healthy.

Discovery of the translocation abnormality in Barbara led to a search for the same abnormality in other members of her family. Tests determined that her mother as well as two aunts and an uncle all had the same balanced-chromosome abnormality. Even more important, the continuing search revealed that four of Barbara's cousins were also balanced carriers of this chromosomal abnormality. Indeed one of the cousins had already had a child with mongolism due to an unbalanced translocation. Another cousin, one of the balanced-translocation carriers, was pregnant at the time. The call from Barbara came in the nick of time. She had an immediate amniocentesis and prenatal study that showed she was carrying a fetus with Down's syndrome, and she and her husband elected to terminate that pregnancy.

After Jim and Barbara had suffered three miscarriages, it was important for them to have chromosomal studies. In about 3 to 8 percent of habitual miscarriages (three consecutive losses), one member of a couple is found to be carrying an abnormal chromosomal pattern. To discover these often subtle abnormalities the use of the new fluorescent chromosome-banding techniques, discussed earlier, is usually necessary. After it was established that Barbara was the carrier of the translocation, the couple wisely availed themselves of the valuable prenatal studies. While their risks of having an affected child were about 10 percent, the knowledge they gleaned from the prenatal studies provided tremendous emotional relief.

Barbara also acted responsibly — and I wish this were the rule — by calling and/or writing to every member of her mother's family. Through her intelligent behavior not only were other carriers detected, but one cousin and her husband were spared the sadness of having a child with serious birth defects.

More Structural Problems

It is possible for a chromosome to break in two places somewhere along its course and the two ends to reattach after turning upside-down (see Figure 8). Since the function of the genes, to some extent at least, may depend upon their position within the chromosome, this process, called *inversion*, may or may not have untoward consequences. Depending upon the chromosome involved, inversion may result in defects such as severe mental retardation, small head (microcephaly), congenital heart disease, and other major birth defects. Inversion may on occasion be hereditary. Other complicated structural abnormalities of chromosomes occur but generally are rare.

Deleted Chromosomes

On occasion a piece of a chromosome may simply break off and disappear: a process called *deletion*. Again depending upon the size of the piece that is missing and which chromosome is involved, various birth defects may occur. The nature of these birth defects may vary from minor to extremely serious. I vividly remember one striking case that occurred when I was working in London, where a deletion had occurred in the #5 chromosome.

Mary, then twenty-seven years old, had sought a consultation with me for a rather unusual reason. She had called the plumber in for repairs two weeks before her consultation. Her baby was then four weeks of age. While repairing her sink in the kitchen, the plumber had asked her if she had acquired a new kitten. She was initially indignant since what the plumber had heard was her baby crying. For the next two weeks, however, her attention began to focus more and more on the baby's cry, which she realized did indeed very much resemble the cry of a cat. Since the baby had also been ex-

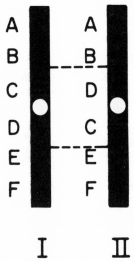

Figure 8 Chromosome inversion showing how a chromosome may break in two places and reattach after turning upside-down.

tremely difficult to feed, she decided that a visit to the doctor was necessary.

She began by complaining about the feeding problem, but it soon became apparent that her main concern was the abnormal cry.

She had had a perfectly normal pregnancy. There was no family history of hereditary diseases.

When I examined the child I found that he was underweight. The cry indeed was remarkably similar to that of a cat. In addition there was a certain roundedness of the face, wide-spaced eyes, and some incurving of the fifth fingers of each hand. A heart murmur was also audible.

The clinical diagnosis I reluctantly and sadly made was the cri-du-chat (cry of the cat) syndrome, which had at that time barely been recognized. Analysis of the baby's chromosomes confirmed the clinical diagnosis and also the poor prognosis of grave mental and physical retardation, which became apparent in the next few months and years.

Broken Chromosomes

Many environmental agents can cause breakage of chromosomes. In 1971 a researcher in Oklahoma first reported breakage in some patients exposed to heavy doses of spray adhesives. This report received national attention and resulted in the almost immediate banning of specific spray adhesives by the United States Federal Drug and Food Administration (FDA). Many laboratories across the United States were deluged with questions concerning the dangers involved in their use as well as requests for chromosomal studies. Because of the preliminary nature of the Oklahoma studies and lack of sufficient normal patients for purposes of comparison, no good guidance could be given to inquiring patients. Many were therefore tested and almost invariably found to have normal chromosomes. In the spring of 1974, the prestigious *New England Journal of Medicine* published a report indicating that no significant chromosomal damage had been noted in a carefully documented study of people exposed to heavy doses of spray adhesives. The FDA subsequently lifted the ban, and there have been no further problems.

Many other environmental agents may cause breakage of chromosomes. A certain amount of x-rays, as used for outlining the intestine (GI series), could cause some breakage of chromosomes in circulating blood cells. Generally this occurrence would be transitory and cause no hereditary problem. However, exposure of a fetus to x-rays could be a serious matter (see Chapter 10). A simple viral infection can also lead to some chromosomal breakage, again with no apparent future ill effects.

Various drugs, including LSD, may cause chromosomal breakage, and these are discussed more fully in Chapter 11.

Virtually all the discussion in this chapter was confined to consideration of the 44 regular chromosomes. Unfortunately, problems with the remaining two sex chromosomes occur even more commonly, and these will form the substance of our next chapter.

CHAPTER 3

Sex Chromosomes

CONTRARY TO SOME EXPECTATIONS the function of the sex chromosomes is to do more than simply "dictate" the sex we become. Problems of sterility, absence or abnormality of menstrual periods, and impotence, to name but a few, may stem from disorders associated with abnormalities of these chromosomes. Indeed, for reasons not understood, abnormality of the sex chromosomes often has a deterrent effect on brain development and function.

As established in Chapter 2, each of our cells contains 46 chromosomes, two of which pertain to sex. We said earlier that the female sex chromosomes are called X, and a woman normally has two of them (XX). The male's sex chromosome is called Y; he normally has one Y and one X (XY) in each cell. However, either male or female may be born with too many X or too many Y chromosomes; also an X or a Y may be missing. The mechanism in the embryo producing this error is the same that occurs with all the other chromosomes and has been described in the preceding chapter.

Individuals possessing a Y chromosome will always appear to be males even if they have two, three, or even four X's as well. A male who appears to have no Y chromosome is an extremely rare exception. Very recent work suggests, however, that this individual probably has a segment of the Y chromosome stuck onto another chromosome, not easily visible, and the power of the sex-determining gene on that tiny piece of the Y chromosome is still operative.

Sex chromosomes can suffer the same breakage or deletion as the other chromosomes. A person can be born with some cells containing normal sex chromosomes and others containing abnormal ones. Such a condition produces what we have already designated as a mosaic individual, a fairly common occurrence for sex-chromosome disorders. Indeed, sex-chromosome abnormalities generally occur at least once in every 500 births!

Too Many Sex Chromosomes

In 1942 research was done on nine male patients who had abnormal breast development, very small testicles, and no sperm production. Certain sex hormones found in the urine were at the high level usually found in castrated males. The body build was feminine and resembled that of the traditional Mid-Eastern eunuch.

This condition is not at all rare, but usually becomes apparent and is diagnosed only after puberty. Males so affected are apt to be taller than the norm and may be intellectually subnormal. A fair number of them fail to adjust to society's written and unwritten standards. Not infrequently they are convicted for petty crimes and sexual offenses and many end up in mental institutions or prisons. Almost every one of them is unable to manufacture sperm.

In 1956, some 14 years after the recognition of the clinical signs of this disorder by Dr. H. Klinefelter, several groups of researchers working in different countries discovered that these males had an extra X chromosome, making their sex chromosome pattern XXY instead of simply XY as in the normal male.

I recall Joey, who was my first patient with the XXY or Klinefelter's syndrome.

Joey, age sixteen years at the time, was brought for consultation by his parents who were concerned because he had been developing rather prominent breasts. They told me that Joey had always been a quiet withdrawn child who seemed to have difficulty getting along with other children, and had emotional and behavioral disturbances both in school and at home. He had been kept back at certain stages of his school career and was now a full three years behind his peers.

He had always grown faster than normal and at the time of the consultation was much taller than boys his own age. The *only abnormal physical sign that the parents mentioned was the curving in of his fifth fingers. My examination revealed also his prominent breasts and rather small testicles. He seemed extremely immature, with borderline intelligence.*

Chromosomal studies showed that he had three sex chromosomes, one of them an extra X. This was an important diagnosis to make since some therapy was available. He was given male hormones as treatment for the rest of his life. The breasts returned quite soon to normal male size. He became slightly more aggressive and able to lead a normal sex life, though he remained sterile.

Individuals born with an extra Y chromosome are of course always male. The XYY syndrome has been associated in the past with a tendency to criminality. This whole matter has generated considerable controversy and will be discussed in detail in Chapter 4.

Truly bizarre sex-chromosome numbers occasionally do occur. For example, there have been persons born with 48 or 49 chromosomes in each cell instead of the usual 46. Women with three X sex chromosomes instead of two may appear physically to be entirely normal and have even incorrectly been called "super-females." The vast majority of these XXX females have no birth defects, but some evidence suggests that a proportion of them suffer from some form of mental disturbance. For example, in a study from Edinburgh, Scotland, of 24 such females after puberty, 22 were found in institutions for the mentally handicapped. Of these, two were classed as feeble-minded, five were schizophrenic, and six had some form of psychosis. While the majority of these so-called triplo-X females appear to be relatively normal — and may even be fertile — behavioral disturbances caused by hidden psychoses can create major problems.

Every now and then women have been found with four X chromosomes instead of two in each cell. Though they seem physically sound and menstruate normally, they have all been severely mentally retarded with I.Q.'s of less than 50.

Too Few Sex Chromosomes

A deficiency of sex chromosomes can also wreak havoc.

A female born with a missing X chromosome will invariably develop into a person with a well-recognized group of physical abnormalities collectively called Turner's syndrome. At birth the infant appears ostensibly as a female, and frequently is noted to have striking puffiness in the back of the hands and feet. This puffiness disappears slowly in the first year of life. In adulthood these women are usually short, under 5 feet, and characteristically have webbing of the neck and a typical facial appearance. While they do develop underarm and pubic hair, their menstrual periods, almost invariably, do not appear. The ovaries are internally underdeveloped, being replaced by a streak of connective tissue. Except for rare exceptions, they are unable to have children. Cyclical estrogen hormones are taken by these patients for breast development and to allow them to have menstrual periods.

It is well known that in between 45 and 60 out of every 100 miscarriages the embryos or fetuses have chromosomal abnormalities. For reasons that are presently still unclear, the commonest abnormality — occurring in about 20 percent of all miscarriages — is Turner's syndrome. It is reassuring that nature is so efficient in ridding the body of abnormal fetuses that only about 2 percent of Turner's syndrome conceptions actually complete pregnancy with a resulting live birth! It is also curious that there appears to be a five- to tenfold increase in twinning among the brothers and sisters of these affected patients. Strangely, too, most of these twins are identical.

Mosaic Chromosomal Patterns

Mosaicism, earlier described as a mixture of cells with normal or abnormal chromosomes, may be extremely difficult to diagnose. Affected individuals vary, depending upon which organs are involved. There are many parents who appear on testing to be completely normal, but have a child with a sex-chromosome problem. Subsequent studies may reveal that one of the parents is a "mosaic" for that particular disorder, who because of the presence of normal cells in vital organs appeared not to be affected.

It can be extremely difficult to confirm a suspected diagnosis of mosaicism. The most common tissues that are studied are blood cells, bone marrow cells, and skin cells. Generally if no mosaic pattern is found in either blood or skin, that person is unlikely to have a mosaic abnormality. It is nevertheless always imprudent to rule out a mosaic pattern in any particular person, since it is conceivable that all cells in blood, bone marrow, and skin may have a normal constitution while the brain cells may have an abnormal set of chromosomes.

There are some other disorders that involve the sex of an individual but are most often not reflected by any abnormality, inherited or otherwise, of the sex chromosomes. In most of those affected something went awry during very early fetal development, when the sex hormones were influencing the formation of the sex organs. Some of these conditions are characterized by unexpected findings, such as apparent *males* with two X chromosomes. This produces an ambiguity that is beset with problems.

It should be made clear at this point that research has not found that homosexuality, transvestism, and other psychological sexual disturbances are due to chromosomal abnormalities or to any other genetic disorder.

The Remarkable Conditions of Intersex

The term *intersex* describes a patient with internal or external genital organs of both sexes. The person may have a penis as well as a vagina and have one ovary and one testis. Abnormalities of the sex chromosomes are not usually associated with these intersex defects. Such individuals may or may not be sterile. Their sexual organs may be infantile and may never mature fully. The penis, for example, may remain the size of a clitoris. Every now and then it is almost impossible to identify the sex of the individual.

True Hermaphrodites

The hermaphrodite, since time began, has been a symbol of tragedy and even of vaudeville humor.

A true hermaphrodite possesses both testicles and ovaries either as two separate organs or as a single combined organ. The external sex organs in these patients vary tremendously and do not help in the diagnosis. They may appear perfectly female, perfectly male, or have external evidence of both male and female sex organs. Most of these patients (and they are rare) have normal female chromosomes. Some, however, have normal male chromosomes, while others are mosaics of mixed female and male chromosome sets. One case history will illustrate the problem:

Rita and Tom had been happy to announce the birth of their first son. At the very first examination after birth, the pediatrician had noted that instead of the hole or meatus being situated at the end of the penis, it was located beneath and at the base of the penis, a condition called hypospadias. One testicle was located in the groin. No other abnormalities were noted and the child underwent surgical repair of his penis. He grew and developed normally and reached puberty without any problems.

At puberty, however, he began to develop very prominent breasts. At the same time the child complained that he was passing blood in the urine for a day or two each month, and the parents brought him in for an immediate consultation.

On examination the boy looked particularly feminine in build with large breasts; the penis was rather small; one testicle was in the groin, and the testicle on the other side did not feel normal and was associated with a groin hernia on the same side.

I suspected an intersex condition and proceeded with various studies. The boy's chromosomes turned out to be female (two X chromosomes). Exploratory surgery later revealed that he had a poorly developed testicle on one side and on the other side, in association with the hernia, a combined poorly developed ovary and testis. In addition he had a small vagina connecting at the base of the bladder, which explained the bleeding in the urine: it was a menstrual period! A tiny rudimentary uterus was connected to the small vagina. The diagnosis of a true hermaphrodite was made on the basis of his having both an ovary and a testis.

Because of the risks of malignancy, both the malfunctioning testis and the ovary plus testis on the other side were removed together with the rudimentary vagina and uterus, and the hernia repaired. The use of male hormones made the breasts regress to normal male size and allowed the boy to continue growing up as a male, albeit sterile.

Pseudohermaphrodites

Unlike true hermaphrodites, pseudohermaphrodites have normal XX or XY sex chromosomes, though their external genital organs tend to resemble those of the opposite sex. Often, as in true hermaphrodites, an abdominal operation is necessary to determine the true condition.

The male has testicles that may, however, be inside the abdomen, stuck in the groin, or even located in the "labia." Frequently these patients, despite their male chromosomes and hidden male organs, have existed and appear as well-developed females who seek medical advice because no menstrual periods have appeared, or because they have had difficulty becoming pregnant. About two-thirds of these patients are likely to have a family history of the same disorder. They may of course not ever have been told about similar abnormalities in other members of the family; indeed, this information has probably been well hidden.

The most common cause of female pseudohermaphroditism (which occurs about 1 in 25,000 births) is a condition called the adrenogenital syndrome. This disorder is inherited from both parents, who are usually normal but carriers of the trait. Generally it is due to an inability of the adrenal gland to manufacture cortisone. At the same time the adrenal gland secretes an excess of a hormone that masculinizes females but has little effect on males. If the lack of cortisone is too severe, it becomes evident in a crisis situation during the second week of life and, if not diagnosed and treated immediately, invariably causes death. If treated promptly, a normal lifespan is possible with permanent daily ingestion of cortisone. There are various types of this disorder, one being associated with high blood pressure.

Masculinization of the female genitals can also be caused when the mother takes certain progesteronelike hormones, usually to prevent threatened miscarriage. The babies when born have normal female chromosomes although the external genitals may appear as male. Treatment with cortisone in these cases is not needed.

The management and treatment of disorders of intersex is a delicate affair. While it might sound logical that a person born with normal female chromosomes should be reared as a female, this is not necessarily always the correct thing to do. More goes into such a decision than simple reliance on the genetic sex of the person. Important factors are 1. what the external sex appears to be; and 2. in what sex the child has been quite naturally reared; and 3. the age at which this diagnostic dilemma arises. Usually it is weeks, months, and sometimes even a few years after birth before the condition is discovered. The general medical recommendation is to allow the child to remain in the sex in which he or she has been reared. Altering the sex is generally considered unwise except in very early infancy. Even then there are parents and doctors who might hesitate. Disorders of intersex cause many severe problems of embarrassment to the individual and family and require the most sophisticated treatment. Severe psychological trauma can be avoided with careful therapy, allowing an afflicted individual to lead a relatively normal though infertile life.

CHAPTER 4

The Myth of the Criminal Chromosomes?

HAS HEREDITY ANYTHING to do with crime, or are all the causes environmental?

Everyone is concerned about the increasing violence in the United States and elsewhere. A multitude of government agencies and many academic scholars of deviant behavior are on the trail of the causes and the solutions. A whole host of social factors is obviously involved: broken homes, child abuse, both psychological and physical deprivation, poverty, overcrowded life in ghettos, and so on. These and other blows of fate on a child may be sufficient cause for the development of criminal or deviant behavior. Yet it is quite possible that a predisposition to mental illness or psychopathic personality may play a strong if not major part.

While it is well known that child abusers are frequently individuals who were abused in their own childhood, there has been no evidence to suggest that the practice is hereditary. Violent crimes may be perpetrated by different members of the same family. Take the case of one Ohio family. When the youngest son was four years of age, his father murdered the boy's mother. As a boy of eighteen, this son also committed murder. Did this boy inherit his father's excessive aggression? Was this simply a coincidental occurrence in the same family? Or was it simply a reflection of early environmental trauma?

The XYY Chromosomal Pattern

Until recently, against this background, the contribution of hereditary factors in causing deviant or criminal behavior has been considered to be generally insignificant. Then in 1961, and quite by accident, the first male with an extra Y chromosome was detected. His blood chromosomes had been studied because he had fathered a child with mongolism. Shortly thereafter research scientists began to wonder whether abnormal sex chromosomes might predispose individuals toward deviant behavior. The idea received international attention in 1965 when Dr. Patricia Jacobs and her colleagues in Edinburgh reported their studies. To determine whether the presence of an extra Y chromosome had anything to do with unusually aggressive behavior, they studied the chromosomes of male patients who were mentally subnormal and being held for treatment in special high security institutions following the commission of various crimes of violence. They found that some 6.1 percent of the 196 males they studied had abnormal chromosomal patterns. Of these males, 3.6 percent had the extra Y chromosome, their sex-chromosomal pattern is therefore called XYY. The investigators were careful to state explicitly that it was not clear whether the XYY males in these high security prisons were antisocial or criminal because of their XYY chromosome constitution, or merely mentally subnormal because of the hormone imbalance.

Characteristics of XYY Males

Men with the XYY sex-chromosomal pattern have in the past been characterized as being of tall stature, with long arms and legs, facial acne, mild mental subnormality, prone to mental illness and to extremely aggressive, dangerous, and antisocial behavior. Such descriptions emanated mainly from studies of prisoners. Only recently, through studying the chromosomes of consecutively born normal male infants and adult males, has it been noted that a very wide spectrum of behavioral and physical characteristics occur in association with the XYY chromosomal pattern. From what is currently known — and a great deal more study is needed — a male with these chromosomes may be entirely normal in all respects, have mild to severe behavioral disturbances, have a borderline normal intellect, or have some nonspecific physical features (e.g., incurved fifth fingers).

Careful studies at the Johns Hopkins University School of Medicine have pointed to a predominance of impulsive acting out in XYY males. These individuals also appear to prefer being alone. No striking abnormality in sexual behavior was evident from these studies.

Boys with the Extra Y Chromosome

Canadian pediatricians and geneticists recently reported a study of four male infants with the extra Y chromosome. None of these children showed any distinctive physical characteristics although three of the four had an unusual feature in their palm prints. The infants were good-looking and had robust physiques. None was particularly tall. One had a severe speech defect. Three of them were perfectly normal in behavior and intellect, neither aggressive, nor destructive, nor hard to manage, but on the contrary pleasant and lovable. One of the children, however, studied at two years nine months of age, showed evidence of aggression and a lack of warm interpersonal relationships with other children. He ate unusual things such as sand or paint chips (a symptom called pica), had diminished language and intellectual ability, and appeared awkward and uncoordinated.

It was possible in this case to interpret his personality defects as originating in his upbringing alone. His extra Y chromosome could have been coincidental. His father was only seventeen years old at the time of his birth and not married to the mother. This seventeen-year-old father also had a retarded sibling and a schizophrenic mother. The child's mother proved to be quite unreliable and wayward, often leaving home without apparent reason and for unknown destinations. The child was reared in this most unstable emotional climate for the first two years and finally in a foster home. In this home they described him as being very stubborn and determined, "like a rock," with an extremely defiant temper "amazing for a two-year-old." He would throw things, bite other children and even adults. He would often eat dirt, gravel, and soap.

Certainly a few of the children with the extra Y chromosome who have been studied have been found to have extremely defiant natures, destructiveness, outbursts of temper when frustrated, and inclinations to climb to dangerous places — all evident by four years of age. Nevertheless, you don't have to be an expert in psychology to recognize that there must be very many children whose behavior is as described but whose chromosomes are normal.

The Extent of the Problem

How many XYY males are born in relation to the whole male population is not yet fully established. From cumulative studies on over 50,000 newborn infants, it appears that about 1 in every 1000 males born has the XYY chromosomal pattern.

Recent studies in the United Kingdom show that the incidence of XYY males among the men admitted to four maximum security institutions in England, Wales, and Scotland in 1972 and 1973 was 2.1 percent. During that two-year period, 70 percent of these XYY males were aged fifteen to twenty years. This meant that 1 in every 16 incarcerated males of that age group had an extra chromosome. A few studies have noted the striking youth (nine or ten years of age) of convicted boys. Careful calculations have suggested that there is a risk of about 1 in 1000 for a normal male being admitted during his lifetime to a high security prison. In contrast, the risk of an XYY male being admitted is 1 percent — at least a tenfold greater risk!

The increased number of XYY males in mental/penal institutions is now well established. What remains entirely unclear is whether the extra Y chromosome has anything to do with it.

Twins and Crime

Some studies on identical and nonidentical twins have shown that in the case of identical twins more often *both* are involved in criminal acts when compared with nonidentical twins. The implication is that some hereditary factor is involved. Unfortunately, however, none of these studies was performed in a way that would take into account familial and environmental factors. Hence no satisfactory evidence can be adduced from these studies to suggest a hereditary criminal factor. The same point is made by a more common example. Consider for a moment families you may know where both children and parents are markedly overweight. Any initial impression that their obesity may be due to familial factors could be readily dismissed after realizing the remarkable quantity of food consumed by the entire family!

Other Chromosomal Abnormalities and Deviant Behavior

It is interesting that surveys done on mentally subnormal, dangerous criminals have shown a higher frequency of males with other sex-chromosome syndromes. A fair number are XXY or even XXYY. Therefore no clear case can be made for singling out the XYY man as the "criminal type," especially when about 11 XYY males, for instance, identified in a survey of French army conscripts and blood donors, were found to have no records of either crime or socially deviant behavior. And in a subfertility clinic in England, seven XYY males were identified who were all respectable law-abiding citizens with no history of mental illness or abnormal behavior.

Restricted Freedom for XYY Males?

Against this background, it is somewhat easier to address a speculation in the *Georgetown Law Journal* in 1969 as to whether society is justified in restricting the freedom of an XYY individual *before* he is proved to have violated the law. Special statutes similar to those in use for "sexual psycho-paths" could be developed to provide indeterminate con-finement without even the necessity of the accused being convicted of a crime — merely being charged with one. From the foregoing, however, it should be clear that the XYY male *cannot* be characterized as a criminal simply by virtue of his chromosomal constitution.

The Prenatal Diagnosis of the XYY Fetus

A few cases have arisen where in the process of prenatal genetic studies aimed, for example, at excluding Down's syndrome an unexpected diagnosis of an XYY fetus has been made. What would you do if suddenly confronted by the news that the fetus you or your spouse carries has been diagnosed as having XYY chromosomes? Would you dwell on the optimistic side believing that there are XYY males without deviant behavior who may lead a perfectly normal life? Or would you believe the present data (yet incomplete) that suggest the eventual risk of committal to a maximum security institution is about 1 in 100? In the few cases with which I am familiar, parents have uniformly elected to terminate such pregnancies in the face of their anxiety and the incompleteness of the available knowledge.

Problems and More Problems

Many major hospital centers, cognizant of the need for more knowledge about the XYY male, initiated large-scale screening studies on newborn infants to determine prospectively not only the incidence of this chromosomal abnormality, but also the development of such offspring. All their studies have been severely criticized, especially the study at one Harvard Medical School hospital, in which the critics concurrently infringed upon the rights of the researchers doing this work. Among the objections raised was that the subjects were inadequately informed before giving consent. The significance of any conclusion made from such a study was also questioned. The criticism that addressed the problem of the so-called self-fulfilling prophecy is important enough to be discussed at length.

The Self-Fulfilling Prophecy

Imagine yourself or your spouse as the parent of a normal-appearing male baby. You had agreed prior to the birth of your son to participate in the newborn-screening program in which a tiny skin prick enables blood analysis of the chromosomes. Unexpectedly chromosomal analysis reveals that the baby has an XYY chromosomal pattern. Would you rather the doctor *not* tell you this information? After all, it is clear from the discussion above that final answers about the ultimate outcome for intellect and behavior of XYY males can still not be forecast with any degree of certainty. Given this real uncertainty, would you and your spouse elect not to have the information?

Your knowledge about your son's abnormal chromosomal pattern may easily influence the way you rear him. For example, knowing his chromosomal abnormality may make you more anxious, more or less demanding of him, insisting on more or less discipline, being more or less permissive, and so on.

Hence, physicians studying such children with an extra Y chromosome may be unwittingly responsible, via the parents, of influencing the child's behavior. Indeed, the criticism goes, this knowledge of the extra Y chromosome may be harmful to the development of the child, as the parents might interpret bad behavioral characteristics as indicative of the child's future criminal disposition and overreact accordingly. For example, a child may enjoy dissecting an insect or even a frog. The parents, knowing about their child's extra Y chromosome, may interpret their son's activity as demonstrating a clear propensity toward murder! A more rational and reasonable explanation would be that he has a well-developed curiosity for biology. Their efforts at disciplining him after such an experience and repeated again in other contexts may destructively influence his childhood years.

If you were about to adopt a child and were informed that he had an XYY constitution, would you complete the adoption process? This possibility is quite real, since in a study at

Johns Hopkins 3 out of 23 XYY males were adopted. Despite problems of the self-fulfilling prophecy, would you insist on knowing this information prior to adoption? In this situation, it would in fact be illegal for this information to be withheld from you — if it were known. As for prenatal diagnosis of the XYY male, it would seem wisest to provide the parents with the most current and accurate information available, while strongly emphasizing the nature and limitations of the available data.

A Plea of Insanity

There have been at least six criminal trials in which the defendant has raised his abnormal chromosomal pattern (XYY) as a basis for a plea of insanity. This defense refers to the legal concept that defines the extent to which accused or convicted individuals may be relieved of criminal responsibility because of mental disease at the time the crime was committed. The defense must first demonstrate that the accused was indeed suffering from a "mental disease." Moreover, a relationship will need to be established between this mental disease and the alleged criminal act.

The insanity defense based on the XYY chromosomal pattern was first raised in April 1968 in France. The defendant, Daniel Hugon, was accused of murdering a sixty-five-year-old prostitute in a Paris hotel. Chromosome studies, made after he attempted suicide, indicated that Hugon had an XYY chromosomal pattern. Nevertheless, he was found legally sane and convicted of murder. The prosecution requested a five- to ten-year sentence rather than the normal fifteen years for similar crimes. Hugon received a seven-year sentence.

In the same year, twenty-one-year-old Lawrence Hannel came to trial in Australia charged with the stabbing death of his seventy-seven-year-old landlady. Again, the same plea of insanity based on his XYY chromosomes was offered. The jury, after only eleven minutes of deliberation, delivered a not-guilty-by-reason-of-insanity verdict, and Hannel was committed to a maximum security hospital until "cured."

Ernest D. Beck, a twenty-year-old farm worker, was tried in Bielefeld, West Germany, in November 1968. The court in this case accepted the prosecution's argument that Beck was fully aware that he was committing murders even though he might not have been able to control his impulses to kill. Beck received the maximum sentence of life imprisonment for the murder of three women.

In April 1969 Sean Farley of New York, a six-foot-eight-inch, twenty-six-year-old male, pleaded not guilty on the grounds of insanity to the alleged brutal murder and rape of a forty-year-old woman in an alley near her home. On cross examination the prosecutor established that it was possible to live a normal life although possessing XYY chromosomes. The jury found Farley guilty of murder in the first degree.

Other convictions have been obtained despite the individual's handicap of having XYY chromosomes. In one celebrated case, Richard Speck, the convicted murderer of eight Chicago nurses, was *incorrectly* characterized as an XYY male. He actually had a normal chromosome constitution!

Because of the difficulties in getting at the truth vis-à-vis the extra Y syndrome, a unique major collaborative study was initiated. Danish and American researchers set out to study, in an unbiased fashion, males with an extra Y chromosome living in the community. They chose Denmark because of the excellent social records kept there.

Tall Men

The researchers decided to study males born in Copenhagen during a particular period, and they chose January 1, 1944, to December 31, 1947, inclusive. Out of a possible 31,436 they were able to account for some 28,884 men, whose heights were also known. They then elected to study only those who were more than six feet tall and were successful in obtaining chromosome analyses on 4139 men.

They found 12 XYY males and 16 males with an extra X chromosome (XXY). Some 41.7 percent of the XYY males and 18.8 percent of the XXY males were found to have been convicted of one or more criminal offenses. This was in contrast to the 9.3 percent figure for males with normal chromosomes. The difference in rates of conviction between the XYY and XXY males was not statistically significant. Moreover, crimes of violence were *not* more frequent among XYY than XXY males, or when compared to males with normal chromosomes (XY).

This study therefore confirmed that XYY males had a higher rate of criminal convictions than normal males, but no greater than XXY males. Both the XYY and XXY males had achieved lower educational levels and had much lower intelligence scores than normal males. No evidence was found to suggest that XYY males were particularly aggressive. Indeed, the essence of the study was the recognition that the antisocial behavior exhibited by XYY males was in all probability a reflection of a low intelligence level, rather than any genetic criminal propensity.

Major Conclusions

There is now little doubt that both XYY and XXY males end up in mental or penal institutions at a higher frequency than XY males. The idea that the extra Y chromosome has a special propensity to induce criminal behavior is a myth that seems to have been exploded. The most likely reason for XYY males ending up in trouble is the low intelligence associated with antisocial behavior. Whether features such as being impulsive, a "loner," prone to an uncontrollable temper, inattention in school, and so on, are symptoms isolated to the XYY syndrome is something that will, we hope, be settled by the awaited second report of the Danish-American study group and by other studies underway.

Meanwhile, what about those parents who discover that they have an XYY male fetus and have to decide for or against abortion? Many are likely to be swayed by the evidence of low intelligence and antisocial behavior; others may take their chances that their son, like some others, will be a normal nonviolent XYY child.

CHAPTER 5

You and Your Genes

THE DISTRAUGHT COUPLE in my consulting room may be disturbed to hear that they both transmitted a harmful gene to their affected child. And what is the difference, they ask me, between genes and this new term, DNA, that crops up all the time in the news? "It is the chemical structure," I answer, "that constitutes the genes."

Reducing our heredity to chemicals is a difficult concept. But it can be understood. The chemicals that make up the universe have been discussed for some time, and it is not a foreign or strange thought that chemicals are the basis of human beings as well as of the atmosphere, rocks, and soil.

Let's make an attempt at this in the area of genetics.

What Are Genes?

Our 46 chromosomes per cell are themselves made up of thousands of tiny pieces, all joined together, not individually visible even under the electron microscope. These submicroscopic pieces are called DNA, the acronym for *deoxyribonucleic acid*, and are very complex structures. These are our genes. They constitute our inherited blueprints that make us what we are physically and mentally.

Each piece of DNA is a tiny, ladderlike structure. The chemicals involved are simple sugars, phosphates, and proteins (see Figure 1). Each rung of the ladder has only two proteins that are linked together chemically in a very precise way. The sides of this ladder are made up of the sugars and the phosphates. In any single chromosome there may be tens of millions of rungs, following each other in a predetermined manner. This predetermined pattern constitutes our blueprint for everything we inherit: color of hair and eyes, shape of

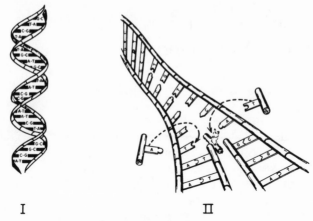

I   II

Figure 1   Structure and Formation of DNA

(I) A strand of DNA made up of many "rungs," representing many
genes. (II) The "copying" or replication process as DNA duplicates
itself. The long twisting DNA strand or "ladder" looks as though it
unzips, chemical substances from the cell joining to form 2 new strands.

nose, type of hair, near- or far-sighted or normal eyes, and so
on, down to the most complicated characteristics that we all
can see, in our relations and friends, passing from generation
to generation.

It has been estimated that a single human cell contains
about 6 million of these DNA rungs. A single gene may con-
sist of perhaps 500 to 2000 rungs on the DNA ladder. The
number of genes contained in a single human cell is still unknown, though generally estimated at between 100,000 and 2.5
million per cell!

For the layman the concept of "gene" and its DNA compo-
nents can be taken together, just as a "sentence" is composed
of "words."

The gene develops by means of the DNA ladder splitting
down the center with chemical substances joining to form two
ladders. The genes function by sending chemical messages to
all parts of the body to influence body growth and the infinite
complex of biochemical functions.

How Genes Are Inherited

Among all these tens of thousands of genes, we could not easily know which "bad" genes we as parents carry, or perceive in our children which parent was responsible for any disease or deformity. Recent scientific advances have made it more possible to find out.

We now definitely know, as discussed in Chapter 3, that we get exactly half our genes from our mother and half from our father. If you have fair skin and suffer badly in the sun it may be a characteristic of only one side of your family. A very high intelligence may be a recognizable family trait: there are some famous cases such as the Darwin family, which produced outstanding scientists for five generations, and the Bernoullis, who generated altogether nine eminent mathematicians or physicists.

On the other hand, genius often springs from completely average families of no particular intellectual distinction, as in the case of Newton, Keats, and Einstein.

Inheriting Harmful Genes from One Parent Only

As we frequently take after one parent more than the other even though we inherit height, hair, and body build genes from both, it can be inferred that the gene we inherited was stronger than its equivalent. Dark hair, for instance, is said to be "dominant." Such dominant genes are harmless, but there are also dominant destructive genes carrying disease or abnormalities (see Figure 2). The parent possessing one will inevitably pass it along to half of his or her children, usually regardless of sex, as in Huntington's chorea (see p. 53). The case history of a family I saw ten years ago gives a good idea of the problem of dominant inheritance.

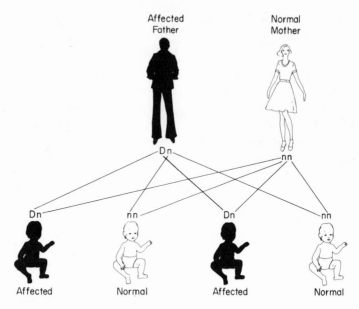

Figure 2   Dominant Inheritance

Above: One affected parent (of either sex) has a defective gene (D) that dominates its normal counterpart (n). Every child has a 50 percent chance of inheriting either the defective gene D (and will then have the disease) or the normal gene n from the affected parent. *Below:* A typical family tree of dominant inheritance, and seen, for example, in Huntington's chorea, heart disease due to hypercholesterolemia, and hundreds of other disorders.

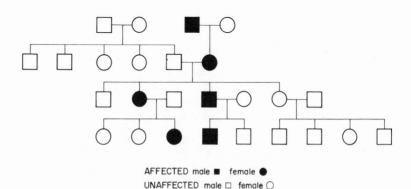

Ann was twenty-one years old, engaged to be married soon. Her father had had some kind of disease affecting the brain and nervous system for some years, the name of which had not been told her. The significance of this disease, unfortunately, had also not been communicated to her. Since the disease was in fact Huntington's chorea, serious questions arose when she became informed of all the facts just a few weeks prior to marriage.

Her fiancé, of course, had not known either that Ann had a 50 percent chance of actually having Huntington's chorea, or that this disease could slowly appear within a few years after marriage. If his wife indeed had the disease (even though it was not yet apparent) and they had children, then there would be a 50 percent risk that each of their children would develop the same disease. In this case, realization of all the facts led the girl's fiancé to break off the relationship and to cancel the marriage. Five years later, sadly, Ann developed Huntington's chorea.

There are hundreds of other dominant diseases. Most circus dwarfs, you will recall, have prominent heads, normal intelligence, and a waddling gait. They have a condition called achondroplasia. This is a dominant disorder. Therefore, should the circus dwarf marry, he or she has a 50 percent risk of having offspring with the same condition. Perhaps you have seen a dwarf of this sort, happily married, to a spouse of normal height, with children who at six years of age are normal and as tall as he or she is. (Many of these achondroplastic dwarfs, incidentally, belong to a famous society called The Little People of America.) It turns out that about seven eighths of these achondroplastic dwarfs have normal parents, which means that this condition can also occur spontaneously, although, as we have already stated, this is a dominantly inherited disorder.

Spontaneous change in the genes, called mutation, can occur, in which a dominant gene is not inherited but created afresh on the chromosome.

Mutation

How does this happen? Earlier we described the gene as a ladder of DNA, which by splitting rungs acts like a mold, allowing, by copying, the formation of identical genes. When some change or fault occurs in this copying process, a gene that is just slightly different is formed. A good analogy is the common experience of taking a key to a locksmith to procure duplicates, only to find that your new duplicate key does not fit the lock properly, although it was copied from the correct key. On your return to the locksmith, he simply files one portion of the key and you return to your lock to discover it now fits perfectly. Of course this simple mechanical correction is not possible for genes, and the mutation is preserved and is copied identically thereafter. Most mutations in human beings occur without known reason. Irradiation either from x-rays, atomic energy, radium, or from the atmosphere is known to cause mutations in genes. This is why it is unwise to irradiate the testes or the ovaries.

Inheriting Harmful Genes from Both Parents

The position of each gene along the length of a chromosome is generally constant and hence a certain function can be mapped more or less accurately at a specific point along one specific chromosome. Every gene for a particular structure or function from one parent is matched with a gene with the same function on the matching chromosome of the other parent. The actual function controlled or directed by the matching genes is a reflection of their *combined* action. If one of the matching genes inherited from one parent is defective, then the other normal gene acts to provide half the needed function, usually enough to keep that person functioning normally. If you are perfectly healthy and free of unusual disorders you might wonder why manifestations of those "four to eight bad genes" you are told you carry are not evident. The answer is that your harmful genes are recessive. The recessive gene has no obvious effect on the body if it has been paired with a normal gene from the other parent, though the genetic function expected from this pair of genes (one defective, one normal) will probably be half of what is normally found. For instance, if the particular gene in question is concerned with the formation and function of a certain enzyme, then it might be possible to demonstrate that you do indeed possess quantitatively only half the strength or activity of that enzyme.

Carriers

If it is found that the activity of a certain enzyme is half of what it should normally be, implying that one of the two genes "controlling" that enzyme is defective, it would mean that you are a carrier of but not a sufferer from the disease that is characterized by virtually no activity of that particular enzyme. Children with Tay-Sachs disease (see Chapter 1) have the enzyme hexosaminidase A missing from their cells, while those who are merely carriers of the disease can be shown to have only half the normal activity of hexosaminidase.

Thus, if your one "harmful" recessive gene is paired with one normal gene, you yourself have no obvious symptoms, but there is a 50 percent chance that each of your children will inherit your defective gene. If you have married a person who has a normal gene of the particular type under discussion, each of your children will also receive one normal gene, and have a 50/50 chance of inheriting two normal genes and of not being a carrier. But most importantly, in this situation, there is no likelihood that any of the children will have two abnormal genes and, therefore, will not develop this genetic disease that is not dominant but "recessive."

If, however, you should marry someone who, like yourself, is also a carrier of the same genetic disease, there is a 25 percent chance in each pregnancy that you will have an *affected* child, a 50 percent chance that a child will also be a carrier like yourselves, and finally a 25 percent chance that a child will not only be entirely normal but not even be a carrier (see Figure 3).

The likelihood that someone who is a carrier of a recessive gene will marry an individual carrying a similar defective gene will vary greatly, depending upon the frequency with which this particular gene occurs in the population at large. For example, approximately 1 in 30 Ashkenazic Jews are carriers of Tay-Sachs disease. Statistically it is possible to calculate — and this has indeed been confirmed — that for about 1 in every 900 Jewish couples, both partners will be carriers. In view of the recessive nature of this disease and the 25 percent chance that this couple may have a defective child, it is possible to calculate that 1 infant in every 3600 live births among Ashkenazic Jews will suffer from Tay-Sachs disease, will appear to develop normally for about the first six months of life, then begin to do poorly, be unable to sit or stand any longer, have seizures, and go blind. Death usually occurs between two and five years of age.

It is obvious, from the small incidence of these recessive diseases, that marriages between two carriers are not common. It is characteristic of recessive hereditary diseases that the genes can pass down through many, many generations without creating any specific family history of the disorder.

Harmful Genes from the Female

It is quite a different story when harmful genes are located on one of the two female sex chromosomes. While many are known to be carried on the female X chromosome, none so far has been discovered on the Y or male sex chromosome. When a female has a harmful gene on one of her X chromosomes, she will pass it along to half her male children and to half her female children (see Figure 4).

The female child who receives the harmful gene from the mother also receives a matching gene that is normal from the father. The effect of the normal gene makes normal (though diminished) function possible, and that female is then only a

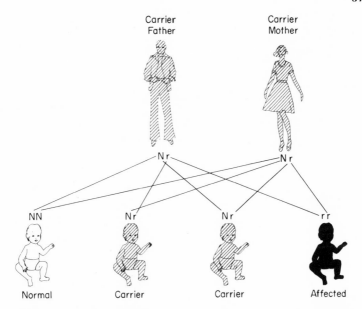

Figure 3   Recessive Inheritance

Above: Both parents are usually healthy, but each carries a defective gene that by itself generally causes no problems. Disease follows when a person receives 2 of these recessive genes. There is a 25 percent chance that a person will inherit a double dose of the defective gene; a 50 percent chance of being a carrier; and a 25 percent chance of being neither a carrier nor affected. *Below:* A typical family tree of recessive inheritance, and seen in cystic fibrosis. Note that there were no previously affected individuals in the family; the cousin marriage is not unusual in such families.

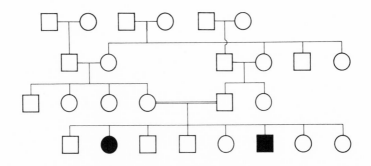

58

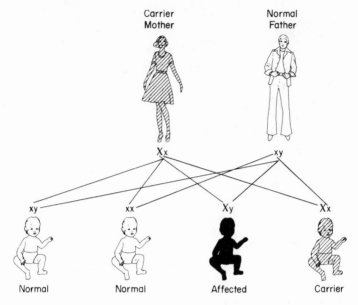

Figure 4 Sex (X)-Linked Inheritance
Above: The defective gene is carried on one X chromosome of the mother, who is usually healthy. Disease follows when that X chromosome containing the defective gene is transmitted to a male. The odds for each male child is 50/50 for being affected, while 50 percent of the daughters will be carriers. *Below:* A typical family tree of X-linked disease such as hemophilia or muscular dystrophy.

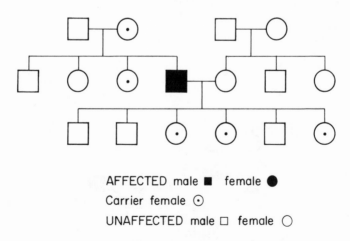

AFFECTED male ■ female ●

Carrier female ⊙

UNAFFECTED male □ female ○

carrier. If one measured the particular enzyme or factor whose deficiency caused a disease, then the carrier would have about half the activity of that enzyme or factor.

One example is hemophilia, a disease of excessive bleeding due to the hereditary absence of one factor that enables blood to clot normally; another is muscular dystrophy, the most common type called Duchenne muscular dystrophy having onset in early childhood with progressive muscle weakness until death usually between ten to twenty years of age.

If you as a female pass along the hemophilia gene to a male child, then he will actually be affected by the disease in question. Since the defective gene you carry is only on one of your two X chromosomes, there is a 50/50 chance your male child will receive the normal one and not even be a carrier (see Figure 4). If, however, the male child inherits the X chromosome with the hemophilia, muscular dystrophy, color blindness gene, or some other sex-linked recessive disease, he will have that condition. If he then marries and has daughters, all of them will receive the X chromosome with the defective gene and therefore become carriers of the disease. Their brothers, because they receive his normal Y chromosome, will neither be carriers nor have the disease (Figure 5). Of course, when an affected male marries a female carrier, the probabilities are quite different (see Figure 6). Note that the commonest condition transmitted on the X chromosome is red/green color blindness: about 8 percent of white males (less in other races) are affected.

Hemophilia is one of the oldest recognized genetic disorders, as there are records in the Talmud dating back before sixth century C.E. The rabbis at the time exempted from circumcision a male child whose brother had bled heavily following this ritual. These exemptions extended to the sons of sisters of a woman who had had a male who bled excessively after circumcision. In their wisdom, this exemption was *not* allowed for the father's son born to other women.

The British royal family provides a typical family "pedigree" for sex-linked disease. Queen Victoria was a carrier of hemophilia, as was her daughter Princess Beatrice. Two of the Princess's sons had hemophilia and one daughter (Queen

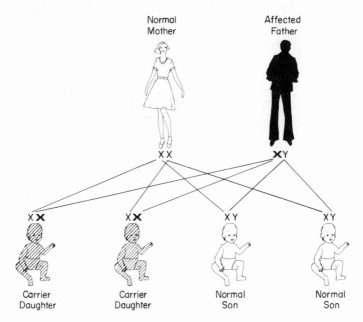

Figure 5 Sex (X)-Linked Inheritance

The defective gene on the X chromosome is on the father's X. He has the disease (e.g., hemophilia). He passes his X chromosome to all his daughters, who become carriers, while none of his sons are affected.

Ena) was a carrier. Queen Ena in turn had two sons who were also affected. And on and on.

There are about 150 diseases transmitted by the sex chromosomes. There are also certain rare hereditary conditions besides hemophilia that are limited to different sexes though the sex chromosomes are apparently not involved. Baldness occurs almost exclusively in males: this is called a sex-dominated trait; and there are some complex disorders that are mainly limited to males or to females.

Mild Symptoms in Carriers

As we have explained, the woman who is a carrier of the gene for a sex-linked disease does not usually have a similar harmful gene on the *other* X chromosome contributed by her unaffected parent. But even with this single dose of the "bad" gene, it would not be remarkable for her to show some mild manifestation of the disease in question. If it is muscular dystrophy, she may well have symptoms of weakness when walking that may become increasingly obvious as she tires during the day. Or, she may have weakness walking upstairs or running for the bus. She or others may have noticed that her calves are seemingly well developed even though she claims that her legs are particularly weak. Likewise the female carrier of hemophilia may not have entirely normal blood-clotting ability. Mothers who are carriers of a white blood cell defect that leads to a disease in which the offspring are especially subject to serious infections (chronic granulomatous disease) can also be shown to have decreased functional ability of their white blood cells to kill bacteria. The mothers of certain albino children may show some pigmentary changes in their eyes.

But it is extremely rare for a female to actually have the sex-linked recessive disease itself. In such cases, the female patient would have to be the daughter of an affected father and a mother who is a carrier, thereby inheriting an abnormal gene from each parent (see Figure 6).

There are some hotly debated data that carriers of the recessive sickle cell anemia may manifest some symptoms of that disease such as higher frequency of strokes caused by hemorrhage or blood clots in the brain or have a diminished life expectancy. A final conclusion on this subject waits for carefully controlled studies made over a long period.

By and large the general rule is that carriers are perfectly normal and healthy and do not realize they are carriers until specifically tested.

There are finally some conditions where the carrier may have greater genetic "fitness" than normal individuals. The now classic example of this greater "fitness" is in the condition mainly affecting blacks for sickle cell anemia. In West Africa, carriers of sickle cell anemia have a higher resistance to the severe form of malaria. Other diseases in which genetic fitness or carrier advantage may occur include the blood dis-

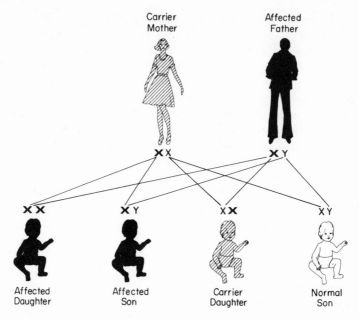

Figure 6 Sex (X)-Linked Inheritance

Above: The defective gene is present on the X chromosome of the father and on one of the X chromosomes of the mother. The father has the disease (e.g., hemophilia) and the mother is the carrier. This time there is a 25 percent chance that a daughter will be affected, and a 50 percent chance for the male to have the disease. *Below:* A typical family tree showing the sequel of a rare marriage between an affected male and a carrier female.

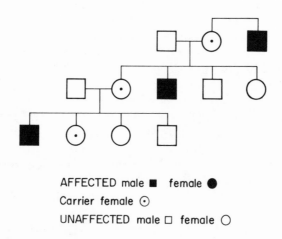

AFFECTED male ■ female ●
Carrier female ⊙
UNAFFECTED male □ female ○

ease called thalassemia, the enzyme deficiency confined to males called glucose-6-phosphate dehydrogenase deficiency, and just possibly cystic fibrosis.

Diseases Limited to Certain Sexes

We have just considered diseases that affect males only (with very rare exceptions), and that are carried by females on their X chromosomes. There are some very rare diseases (e.g., Vitamin D Resistant Rickets) that affect only one of the sexes, but that are *not* transmitted via the sex chromosomes.

The critical distinguishing characteristic of sex-linked dominant inheritance is that an affected male transmits the harmful gene to *all* his daughters but to *none* of his sons. As for other dominant type diseases, marked variability, called heterogeneity, of the disease may be found in the person with the defective gene. The effects will vary from remarkably mild, to severe, to fatal.

Genetic Disease Caused by Multiple Factors

There are many elements, not the least being the environment, that combine with minor gene abnormalities to produce serious defects. It is not really understood how environmental factors operate, but the correlation of many common diseases with geography and social conditions is obvious. In this category we find cleft lip and palate, club feet, congenital hip dislocation, spina bifida (open spine) and anencephaly (brain defect), some congenital heart defects, and possibly predisposition to coronary artery disease, certain types of diabetes, hypertension, and allergies — to name but a few.

The environmental causation is linked in some way to the genetic tendency. We find that seasonal clustering is especially characteristic of some of these diseases such as anencephaly (which especially affects babies born in autumn and winter), dislocation of the hips, and certain heart defects (including patent ductus arteriosus, coarctation of the aorta, and ventriculoseptal defect). German measles (rubella) may account for some of these defects, as well as widespread viral infections in a community at a certain time. In fact, virtual epidemics of anencephaly in the newborn have been recorded in New England, strongly suggesting the action of a virus.

Geography must play its part when you consider that in Great Britain alone the incidence of spina bifida and anencephaly falls dramatically as one moves from Northern Ireland to the south of England: 7 in 1000 births in Belfast reduce to about 2 per 1000 in southern England. The effect of the original homeplace on groups of people seems to remain even when they move to a drastically different locale; the Irish in Boston have kept their higher risks of spine and brain defects.

Economic conditions play a still unconfirmed role, though it is well recognized that poorer whites suffer a higher frequency of nervous system malformations at birth. Yet blacks in the United States have a low incidence of these malformations, just as they do in West Africa and in Great Britain, in spite of their generally disadvantaged condition. The higher frequency of these conditions in the Sikhs in the Punjab is also reflected in births to Indians and Pakistanis (also mostly from the Punjab) in certain areas of England. Some preliminary data suggest that Irish women married to black West Indian husbands still have a higher frequency of births with these brain and nervous system defects.

Finally, both maternal age and birth order are factors influencing the birth of babies with spina bifida and anencephaly. The first-born and the fourth and later children in a family are most in danger. Mothers under twenty and over thirty-five seem to have defective children in excess of those in the middle range of their reproductive life.

In general, for these so-called polygenic disorders that we have been discussing, the general risks of recurrence to parents who have already had one such child is 3 to 5 percent in every subsequent pregnancy. If they have been so unfortunate as to have had two such affected children, the risks rise to somewhere between 8 and 12 percent. It should be noted that if one parent was born with such a defect, the couple has a 3 to

5 percent risk in the very first pregnancy. There is also about an eightfold increase in the occurrence of open spine defects among the first cousins of affected individuals (see Chapter 9).

There are then, in essence, three different categories of hereditary disease. The first type, discussed in Chapter 2, concerned abnormal chromosomes: either in number or structure. The second group of genetic disease is related to harmful genes that we inherit or that occur through mutation causing recessive, dominant, or sex-linked diseases. The last group is the one we've just discussed: disorders that reflect the interaction of specific genes with certain as yet unrecognized agents in the environment.

Mild to Severe Disease

Analysis of the pattern of inheritance from the family pedigree can be most confusing. One reason may be that the "bad" gene may not always be expressed to the same degree as it was in the parent from whom it came. For example, there is a dominant hereditary disorder that affects the brain and nervous system called neurofibromatosis. The affected person may have birthmarks on the skin that look like coffee stains, soft little lumps along the course of nerves, and possibly larger tumors originating from nerves in any organ such as the brain, kidney, or lung. Because the gene for this disorder may vary in its strength of expression, one might find that the parent simply has a few typical marks on the skin, while the affected children (50 percent of the offspring would be affected) would have not only the birthmarks, but also multiple tumors, leading perhaps even to early death because of the site of these tumors. While these variations in gene expression are more often and easily perceived in the hereditary *dominant* disorders, it is not unusual to find also variability in the recessive disorders. Out of several children in the same family with albinism, some may have complete and others partial involvement. In cystic fibrosis, one sibling may be more severely affected than another, and so on.

Awareness of this possible variation in gene expression is

important in interpreting family pedigrees. Occasionally, it might be thought either that there is no family history whatsoever for a particular disorder or that a generation was skipped. It is therefore important always to be certain that the allegedly unaffected individual has indeed no sign of the disease. Such certainty may only be possible after actual physical examination of or special tests on the parents or close relatives.

There is another dominant hereditary disease called tuberous sclerosis, where the affected person may have an acnelike rash over and around the nose and cheeks, mental retardation, epileptic seizures, tumors of muscle (especially heart), as well as tumors behind the eye. When a child is born with signs of this disease, the parents should automatically be examined because of the dominant mode of inheritance in about 50 percent of these cases (the other 50 percent arise spontaneously due to mutation). Careful physical examination of both parents may reveal no signs of the disease, and the false conclusion of a mutation could be made. However, this kind of conclusion can only be safely made after extensive and careful study including x-rays of the skulls of both parents as well as x-rays of the chest, kidneys, and so on. The reason for this very critical examination is that the risk of recurrence will be zero if both parents are genetically normal, but 50 percent if one parent is found to have some sign of the disease.

The Time of Onset

One of the most intriguing aspects of genetic disease relates to the age of onset of a particular disorder. There are many variations. A child born with muscular dystrophy of the sex-linked variety (males only), as mentioned earlier, may appear to be entirely normal during the first one to five years of life. Children born with Tay-Sachs disease appear perfectly normal at birth and for the first five to six months of life. But from the first day of life — indeed from the twelfth week (or earlier) of fetal life — a certain biochemical enzyme deficiency can be demonstrated. Some hereditary disorders may not become apparent until forty to sixty-five years of age, such as Huntington's chorea, though there may be clinical signs discernible at age fifteen.

Many of these observations really make you think about the factors that govern our normal development. Why, for example, does puberty occur when it does? What conditions our growth spurt? What "body clock" mechanism causes the menopause? Why do some people become diabetic late in life? Historically, much of the research on rare genetic diseases has shed unexpected light on normal body processes, such as aging, and the function of many genes.

Clearly, then, we all have harmful genes, which are inherited from one of our parents or originate at our conception. It is already possible — and it will become more common — to determine which harmful genes we carry. There are some good reasons why you should be concerned and they form the substance of the next two chapters.

CHAPTER 6

Genes, Race, and Relatives

PERHAPS SOME OF US would like to think of ourselves as being different — and indeed we are — though all members of the human species. The first major difference is our racial origin. Three distinct groups are easily distinguishable: African (black), Caucasian (white), and Oriental (yellow). Representatives of all three today inhabit every continent, and, over the centuries, very significant mixing has occurred. It is easy to distinguish a person's race when the color differences are really striking, but mixing has tended to make it harder and harder to determine the origins of some people. Study of the differences between gene effects has been useful in this regard. It has become clear, however, that genetic differences between races appear small in comparison to those between the ethnic groups within races.

A few genetic characteristics, such as certain blood groups, even used alone, may indicate an individual's ethnic group. Africans virtually all have the so-called Duffy blood group, in contrast to only 3 percent of whites with this genetic marker. Rh negative blood occurs rarely among Africans, and is most frequent in whites; and there are other genetic markers that give us clues that allow differentiation of racial groups.

The Gene Advantage

Possession of certain genes by people living in defined areas of the world has proved to be beneficial to their health. This advantage has best been shown for sickle cell anemia (a progressive, hereditary, and ultimately fatal hemolytic anemia), which mostly affects blacks, Greeks, and Asiatic Indians causing about 100,000 deaths yearly. Many years ago it was noticed that in areas where malaria was rife, there was also a high frequency of sickle cell anemia. Ultimately it was clearly shown that those individuals carrying the gene for sickle cell anemia were much more resistant to malaria. You will recall that sickle cell anemia is a recessive disorder, and the gene is carried equally by both parents. While the individual affected by this anemia is ill, the carriers are not. Indeed carriers turn out to have an advantage or be "fitter," in that they are able to resist malaria much better than those of us without the sickle cell gene.

Other genetic adaptations to disease are known that also confer advantages on the bearer of the specific gene. Thalassemia, for example, is a fatal, hereditary anemia similar to sickle cell anemia (involving changes in bones and skin and spleen enlargement) found mainly in people who live in or originate from the Mediterranean region: especially Italians and Greeks, as well as Africans and Indians. Again carriers are more resistant to malaria. Female carriers of the sex-linked enzyme disorder called glucose-6-phosphate dehydrogenase are more resistant to malaria; this disorder also occurs in those who live in the malarial belts of the world.

One highly speculative and unproven selective advantage was suggested for Tay-Sachs disease. It was thought that carriers were more resistant to tuberculosis, a disease that was rife in the overcrowded ghettos of Eastern Europe, from which these carriers probably originated.

Genes and Climate

It may have occurred to you that skin color (determined by your genes) is closely related to areas where there is much sunshine. The closer to the equator, the stronger the sunlight, the more likely the skin will be dark. Hair and eye color (both gene determined) have similar distributions to skin color. Dark-colored skin, eyes, and hair are advantageous in hot, bright climates.

The so-called peppercorn hair of Africans may prevent

rapid evaporation of sweat, possibly protecting their heads from excessive heat and sunstroke. The absence of facial hair on Orientals originating in northern and eastern climes has been considered an advantage in preventing frostbite. The narrow eyes and the eye-fold near the nose in Orientals may protect the eye from the elements. Since body heat is retained better by larger bodies, it should come as no surprise to you, at this stage of the discussion, to discover that body size increases with latitude! So much for gene advantages. Let us move on to what is perhaps more common — disadvantageous genes.

Genes in Isolation

Many populations in the world have among them groups of people who isolate themselves from the rest on religious or other grounds. Such a group may remain as an "isolate" for many generations, inbreeding being the expected and actual consequence, with more and more sharing the same harmful genes they have inherited. The children born in any isolated group show the manifestations of inbreeding by virtue of an increased frequency or unusual nature of birth defects or genetic disorders.

Isolated Alpine villages are known where the frequency of albinism is high. Other villages have high rates of deaf-mutism, blindness, or mental retardation. On one Pacific Ocean atoll, Pingelap, about 5 percent of the population are totally colorblind (achromatopsia), a condition that is associated with severe nearsightedness and other serious eye problems. In one community of the Amish in Pennsylvania, a particular type of dwarfism with extra digits has been recognized. The Amish — a religious and social isolate — intermarry, and few genes from the "outside" are ever added to the community.

Ethnic groups, to an extent, represent genetic isolates because of inbreeding. Let us explore the consequences of our ethnic origins.

Hereditary Disease and Ethnic Group

The chances that a child of yours will suffer from or carry a hereditary disorder may in large part be due to your ethnic origins (Tables 1, 2, and 3). The high frequency of some diseases (Tay-Sachs disease, familial dysautonomia) that are found among Ashkenazic Jews is not seen in Sephardic Jews. While familial Mediterranean fever may be common in Sephardic Jews, it is rarely found in Ashkenazic Jews.

Blacks in the United States carrying the sickle cell gene brought it with them from Africa. Now some 1 in 10 black Americans are carriers of this disorder, and a child with sickle cell anemia occurs in about 1 in 400 black births.

Cystic fibrosis is the most common genetic killer of white children. About 1 in every 2500 are born with it, and 1 in every 25 whites is a carrier. Cystic fibrosis in blacks or Orientals is positively rare. When it does occur, it is almost invariably related to white admixture somewhere in the family history. Phenylketonuria (PKU), a hereditary biochemical disease causing mental retardation when untreated, similarly is mostly found in whites and is rare in blacks and Orientals.

It should be clear that any of these diseases could occur, through intermarriage or mutation, in any ethnic group. (Tay-Sachs disease is found in children who are not Jewish, even though it is at least 100 times less frequent.) Questions about an individual's country of origin or ethnic group, therefore, can be crucial in alerting the physician to the diagnosis of a rare and unsuspected disease. A recent example illustrates this point:

Pietrus was a twenty-four-year-old, married graduate student who came to the emergency ward complaining of severe abdominal pain and vomiting. His symptoms began on the very day that he came to the hospital; he said that up to that day he had been in excellent health except for some constipation, though he admitted to one previous similar episode that had also landed him in the hospital and resulted in the re-

Table 1   Some Genetic Disorders in Different Ethnic Groups*

Ethnic Group	Genetic Disorders
Africans	Hemoglobinopathies, especially Hb S, Hb C, alpha- and beta- thalassemia, persistent Hb F
	Glucose-6-phosphate dehydrogenase deficiency, African type
	Adult lactase deficiency
Afrikaners (South Africans)	Variegate porphyria
Armenians	Familial Mediterranean fever
Ashkenazic Jews	Abetalipoproteinemia
	Bloom's syndrome
	Dystonia musculorum deformans
	Familial dysautonomia
	Factor XI (PTA) deficiency
	Gaucher's disease (adult form)
	Iminoglycinuria
	Meckel's syndrome
	Niemann-Pick disease
	Pentosuria
	Spongy degeneration of brain
	Stub thumbs
	Tay-Sachs disease
Chinese	Thalassemia (alpha)
	Glucose-6-phosphate dehydrogenase deficiency, Chinese type
	Adult lactase deficiency
Eskimos	E_1^s (pseudocholinesterase deficiency)
Finns	Congenital nephrosis
	Aspartylglucosaminuria
Irish	Neural tube defects
	Phenylketonuria
Japanese and Koreans	Acatalasia
	Oguchi's disease
	Dyschromatosis universalis hereditaria
Mediterranean peoples (Italians, Greeks, Sephardic Jews)	Thalassemia (mainly beta)
	Glucose-6-phosphate dehydrogenase deficiency, Mediterranean type
	Familial Mediterranean fever
	Glycogen storage disease, Type III
Norwegians	Cholestasis-lymphedema
	Phenylketonuria

* This table simply provides you with a perspective of the extent of hereditary ethnic disorders. Any specific concern is best discussed with your doctor.

Table 2   Selected Genetic Disorders in Some Ethnic Groups

If You Are	The Chance Is About	That
black	1 in 10	You are a carrier of sickle cell anemia
	7 in 10	You have an intolerance to milk (e.g., develop diarrhea)
black and male	1 in 10	You have a hereditary predisposition to develop hemolytic anemia after taking sulfa or other drugs
black and female	1 in 50	
	1 in 4	You have or will develop high blood pressure
white	1 in 25	You are a carrier of cystic fibrosis
	1 in 80	You are a carrier of phenylketonuria
Jewish (Ashkenazic)	1 in 30	You are a carrier of Tay-Sachs disease
	1 in 100	You are a carrier of familial dysautonomia
Italian-American or Greek-American	1 in 10	You are a carrier of thalassemia
Armenian or Jewish (Sephardic)	1 in 45	You are a carrier of familial Mediterranean fever
Afrikaners (white South African)	1 in 330	You may have porphyria
Oriental	Close to 100%	You will have milk intolerance as an adult

moval of his appendix. This had been some five years ago, and he reported that the doctor had said after the operation that the appendix had, surprisingly, looked perfectly normal. No family history was available, since he had been adopted.

General physical examination revealed a well-built young man with only slight fever, persistent vomiting, dehydration, and complaints of severe abdominal colic with only some abdominal tenderness.

A series of blood tests followed by x-rays still did not reveal the cause of his abdominal pain, and questions began to arise about the possibility of poisoning. An alert young physician noted that Pietrus had been born in South Africa, which prompted him to suggest a urine test to exclude a condition that has a mortality rate of about 24 percent with acute at-

**Table 3   The Frequency of Some Genetic Diseases
in Certain Ethnic Groups**

If You Are	The Chance That Your Child Will Have*	Is About
black	Sickle cell anemia	1 in 400
	Thalassemia	8 in 1000
white	Cystic fibrosis	1 in 2500
	Phenylketonuria	1 in 25,000
Jewish (Ashkenazic)	Tay-Sachs disease	1 in 3600
	Familial dysautonomia	1 in 10,000 to 20,000
Italian-American or Greek-American	Thalassemia major	1 in 400
Armenians or Sephardic Jews	Familial Mediterranean fever	1 in 8000

* These approximate risk figures apply only if both you and your spouse are of the same ethnic group.

tacks. This condition, correctly considered and diagnosed by the young resident, was acute intermittent porphyria, a complex, hereditary biochemical disease of proteins that affects the nervous system and other organs, which indeed is common in South Africans of Dutch descent. He probably inherited the gene for this dominant genetic disease from one of his parents. This recognition was important not only in saving the patient from additional surgery, but it also alerted him never to allow himself to be given barbiturates for any reason, since barbiturates often cause severe attacks and may prove fatal to porphyria patients. Moreover, he then received careful genetic counseling during which it was explained that he and his wife had a 50 percent risk in every pregnancy of having an affected child. He elected to have a vasectomy and the couple adopted first one and then a second child.

Extensive and laborious studies by Dr. G. Dean, in South Africa, established that porphyria was introduced there by a pair of immigrants from Holland who married there in 1688. Today about 1 in 330 white South Africans actually possess the gene for porphyria and are affected by this disease. Because anesthesia, barbiturates, and even other drugs may prove fatal to affected individuals, many hospitals in South Africa actually do tests routinely for this disease on every patient on admission.

The Genes and History

Why, you may have wondered, should a disorder such as Tay-Sachs disease be carried by about 1 in 30 Ashkenazic Jews regardless of where they live? The same question could be asked for various other diseases that especially affect certain ethnic groups (see Table 1). The most likely and obvious explanation is that these individuals have a common ancestry and therefore may share the same "bad" genes. Their dispersion across the globe as mirrored by historical events serves to explain why they are afflicted by the same genetic diseases that are quite different from those of Sephardic Jews. It seems that Ashkenazic Jews descended from those who fled to Northeastern Europe after the sacking of Jerusalem by the Romans in 70 c.e. The Sephardim (Oriental or Spanish Jews) are probably descended from those who fled to Babylon after the destruction of their first temple in 586 b.c.e. The Jews in Iran and many of those now in Israel are the likely descendants of these exiles, as are those who fled eastward from the Romans in 70 c.e. to North Africa and Spain. Subsequent changes in the genes from mutation and inbreeding probably largely explain the occurrence of certain different diseases in these two groups of Jews as well as the frequency with which they occur.

Through blood group studies, it has been possible to come to some conclusions about the movement of the Celts, who include peoples of Cornish, Welsh, Irish, and Scottish descent and the Vikings of Norway (Norsemen). The Vikings invaded Ireland and Britain and temporarily settled there until their final eviction in the late tenth and early eleventh centuries c.e. Some Norsemen, after leaving Ireland and Britain, settled in Iceland, taking with them Celtic wives and slaves. Genetic evidence shows that most of the early settlers in Iceland were Celts rather than Norsemen. The genetic evidence is based on the peculiar frequency of specific and different blood group systems in peoples of those areas today. From similar studies it has been deduced that there is a common ancestry for inhabitants of the west coasts of Norway, Scotland, and Ireland. The most likely explanation appears to be the importation of Celtic women as wives and slaves of Norsemen to Norway in the Viking period.

Scholars have long pondered the origin of the European Gypsies. The majority of these gypsies once lived in Hungary, as isolated groups in which there was much inbreeding. It has been noted that a remarkable difference exists between the frequencies of the ABO blood group system in Gypsies compared to Hungarians. The blood group systems in Gypsies, however, are remarkably similar to those in Asiatic Indians and it is thus probable that the Gypsies have Indian origins.

Blood Groups

Each of us possesses different genes that control the development of different blood group or protein substances. The ABO blood group system was discovered by Dr. Karl Landsteiner in 1900. Your blood group is determined as A, B, O, or AB (and there are many others) by virtue of specific proteins coating the surface of red blood cells. Since 1900, some 250 different proteins on and in the red blood cell alone have been recognized. Correctly matching blood is therefore critical before blood transfusions are given.

Not unexpectedly, ethnic differences occur in the frequency of blood groups. The B gene, for example, is three times more frequent in Orientals than in whites, whereas in virtually all American Indians the B gene is almost entirely absent.

The Rh blood groups were discovered in 1939, and are thus named because the blood of rhesus monkeys was used in the experiments. Persons having the specific Rh protein or antigen are Rh positive, characterizing about 84 percent of all

Caucasians; the other 15 percent do not have this protein and are called Rh negative.

If an Rh negative woman becomes pregnant by an Rh positive man, and this really is the main hazard, then the fetus may be Rh positive. In such a case the Rh antigen crosses over into the fetus, whose body recognizes the foreign protein and counters by making a protein antibody to "fight" the "invader." This newly made antibody recrosses into the mother's blood and remains there permanently. In the first pregnancy usually no problems occur. However, with the mother sensitized by the fetal antibody, in the second and subsequent pregnancies it crosses the placenta and begins a process of destroying the red blood cells and tissues of each Rh positive fetus. Fetal death, stillbirth, or severely ill newborns with anemia and jaundice may be the result. Blood transfusion of the fetus in the womb or exchange transfusion after birth may be lifesaving, and also prevent later mental retardation. Note that an Rh negative mother may become sensitized from a previous incompatible blood transfusion, which would affect the very first pregnancy. Similarly, sensitization of the mother may occur during an unrecognized miscarriage, very early in pregnancy. Then in the second pregnancy, which she thinks is her first, the fetus may be affected.

It is obviously of the greatest importance, to you and to every couple who plans to have a child, not only to know your genes but to find out your Rh group. The reason is that due to continuing advances in medical research it is now possible to prevent an Rh negative woman from becoming sensitized simply by having an injection of a specific protein, immunoglobulin, at the birth of her first baby. Because of these advances, jaundice in the newborn is steadily being wiped out. Remember, however, to find out your (and your spouse's) Rh group before pregnancy; and ensure that the first visit to the doctor does not occur when pregnancy has already progressed some three to four months.

In addition to red blood cells, other inherited blood group systems have been sought and found that vary among individuals. Over 30 different antigens can be detected on white blood cells. This group constitutes what is called the HL-A system: one that is crucial to the careful matching necessary for organ transplantation.

Many other specific proteins occur in the blood serum and allow for more exact individuation.

Blood Groups and Disease

The search for associations between ABO blood groups and disease has been relatively unrewarding. Perhaps the most firmly established association is between blood group O and duodenal ulcer. Even then, Type O occurs only about 1.4 times more often in people with duodenal ulcer. Pernicious anemia and stomach cancer are slightly more common in those of Type A blood, while stomach (as opposed to duodenal) ulcers are a little more common in Type O individuals. Type A is associated with a rare birth defect called the Nail-Patella syndrome characterized by either total absence (or abnormalities) of nails and absent or defective kneecaps. A dominantly inherited muscle disease, myotonic muscular dystrophy, is associated with another blood group system called the Secretor system.

Incompatibility between mother and baby in the ABO blood groups only occasionally causes problems (anemia and/or jaundice) after birth.

There is a recent interesting observation that suggests that young women taking oral contraceptives have a higher incidence of blood clotting complications if they have Type A, B, and AB than those who have blood group O.

HL-A Proteins and Disease

The search for specific disease associations between the unique HL-A antigens on white blood cells has been more fruitful. In the HL-A system, the various proteins are numbered and of course are controlled by different genes. Without going into unnecessary detail, it is sufficient for our purposes here to note that some clear associations have emerged. A form of rheumatoid arthritis affecting the spine, called ankylosing spondylitis, has been correlated with an HL-A protein called B27. About 90 percent of persons with this protein have the disease, though this B27 protein occurs in only 7 percent of the European population. Hence, finding it present is an aid to diagnosis. Psoriasis is associated with HL-A groups 13, 16, and 17; celiac disease with B8; insulin-dependent diabetes with A8 and W15, and multiple sclerosis with A3, B7, and DW2. Thus far a variety of other correlations have been noted, but are less strong. We are talking here only about strong correlations and not saying that someone with a particular inherited protein group will definitely develop a certain disease. These associations do imply, however, that there is a genetic component to these diseases.

Consanguinity and Incest

As far as harmful genes are concerned, as said earlier, all of us are carriers of four to eight "bad" genes. For the most part they have little effect on our health or that of our offspring. It has been estimated that about one in three of us carries a gene for severe mental defect. As we have demonstrated, when we marry and procreate with someone of the same ethnic group (e.g., Celt with Celt, Jew with Jew, and so on) then the chance that we have the same harmful gene in common rises significantly. Taking this one step further, it should be clear that if close relatives like first cousins marry, called consanguinity, they are even more likely to have harmful genes in common and therefore would have a slightly increased risk of having genetically defective offspring. Because first cousins have two grandparents in common, it can be calculated that their risk of having a child with a birth defect would approximate 6 to 8 percent in each pregnancy. This would be in contrast to the known 3 to 4 percent incidence of serious birth defects or mental retardation in the population at large. First cousins thus have a risk about double that of the average couple. While it is known that first cousin marriages are noted more frequently among the parents of mentally retarded individuals, they nevertheless do have a better than 90 percent chance of having normal offspring.

Many countries and at least half the United States prohibit marriages between uncle-niece, aunt-nephew, as well as between first cousins. In contrast, the latter is actually encouraged in some societies, as in certain areas of Japan where 10 percent of marriages occur between first cousins. In one state of India, Andhra Pradesh, uncle-niece marriages are encouraged, and such unions may constitute about 10 percent of all marriages in the area. In uncle-niece or aunt-nephew marriages, a threefold increase in birth defects would be expected.

Based on the above calculations and remarkably little good data, most countries prohibit marriage between relatives as close as first cousins. In the United States less than 1 in 1000 marriages are between first cousins. Though the highest reported rate of marriages between relatives is found in Japan (4 in 100 marriages), in certain isolated groups around the world the rate of marriage between relatives may be as high as 25 percent! As far as the genes go, such marriages in these lonely communities reduce the number of carriers but increase the number of offspring with genetic disease.

Intercourse between brothers and sisters, fathers and daughters, mothers and sons, constitutes incest and is not only illegal but considered taboo in most societies. The reported studies of incest all note a devastating increase in the occurrence of serious birth disorders and/or mental defects. Such unions would be expected to result in about a fivefold increase in the birth of defective offspring.

Rape and Murder

I hope it has become clear now that the uniqueness of an individual can be established biochemically by measuring not only the blood group, but also by assessing exactly other genetically transmitted proteins found on the surface of and within the red and white blood cells, in the bloodstream (serum), and in various body secretions such as saliva or semen. There are literally hundreds upon hundreds of different proteins that can be utilized when there is a specific need to identify a particular person. For the red blood cell alone, more than 250 different proteins have been recognized. Hence, in cases of murder or rape, examination of a tiny speck of blood (and remember you cannot even see a single red blood cell with the naked eye) or some semen can rapidly assist in the identification of a suspect, and the fruits of genetic research have become important in the solution of crimes of rape and murder. The accurate distinction now possible between human beings on the basis of various genetic blood tests has made identification almost as certain as fingerprinting! When one adds the unique characteristics of individual chromosomes when specially stained (see Chapter 2, p. 14), we are generally in an extremely strong position to verify a murder or rape suspect.

And Who Is the Father?

Nowadays court proceedings involving disputed paternity are not unusual. The various blood group systems and the chromosomes both provide extremely valuable information. The courts have and still tend to use this information to show that the man disputing that he is the father could not be the real father, rather than trying to prove someone else is the father. For example, a man is excluded as the father if both he and the mother lack a specific blood group that the child has. The child cannot, of course, have a blood group that both parents lack. A variety of possible blood groups in children from marriages between individuals with known ABO blood groups is shown in Table 4.

The uniqueness then, of each human inheritance is such that even given the same blood group system on our red blood cells, we invariably differ with regard to other body proteins on white blood cells, platelets, serum, and so on. It is easy to understand why transplanting a kidney or other organs from a donor to an ill person is fraught with the difficulty of making

Table 4   Problems of Disputed Paternity*

1 Blood Groups at Marriage			2 Possible Blood Groups of Children	3 Blood Groups That Are Impossible in Children of This Marriage
One Partner	×	Other Partner		
O	×	O	O	A, B, AB
O	×	A	O or A	B, AB
O	×	B	O or B	A, AB
O	×	AB	A or B	O, AB
A	×	A	O or A	B, AB
A	×	B	O or A or B or AB	None
A	×	AB	A or B or AB	O
B	×	B	O or B	A, AB
B	×	AB	A or B or AB	O
AB	×	AB	A or B or AB	O

* The ABO blood group system shows various marriage combinations with the possible blood groups of their children. It would be impossible for the father (either partner in column 1) to have sired a child whose blood group appears in column 3.

a correct match-up. We have all heard about the rejection by an ill and needy body of the organ donated. Dramatic advances have been made in this field of blood and tissue matching — called histocompatibility testing — and such progress can be expected to continue.

CHAPTER 7

The Gene Screen

MOST OF US do not know which harmful genes we carry. If we have a child with a hereditary disease, we know — at least for one gene. If a close relative is affected, we should be alerted to have special tests. The first clue may, however, be too late to avert tragedy. Advances in medical technology enabled for the first time all newborns to be tested for certain genetic disorders causing mental retardation. More recently programs have been developed to determine carriers of specific genetic disorders in various ethnic groups at risk, thereby alerting couples to other options prior to the conception or birth of a defective child.

Screening for Harmful Genes

The screening of newborns has been adopted worldwide for obvious reasons. Early detection has allowed for the initiation of early treatment and the prevention of mental retardation in a few of the hereditary disorders, such as phenylketonuria (Chapter 22), and most recently of hypothyroidism (deficient thyroid hormone production resulting in mental retardation if not treated soon after birth). There have been few objections to such programs except perhaps to their overall cost. Screening newborn babies for chromosomal disorders has in comparison aroused controversy for a number of reasons including the absence of a specific treatment.

Screening programs to detect carriers have also caused some doubts and objections, which I referred to in Chapter 5. Only two such major population screening programs have been tried, one for Tay-Sachs disease among those of Jewish descent, and one for sickle cell anemia carriers in the black community. Such programs, to succeed, involve a number of critical though minimal prerequisites including:

1. Definite knowledge about the pattern of inheritance for that particular disease; e.g., if the disease to be tested is recessive, both parents must be carriers.
2. An available, well-defined ethnic community with a higher risk for the particular disease that is being screened.
3. An accurate, reliable, rapid, simple, automated, and inexpensive method of detecting individuals who carry these disorders.
4. The possibility of diagnosing the actual disease in the fetus so that couples who are both found to be carriers can elect to prevent serious or fatal genetic disease through prenatal diagnosis, early treatment where possible, or pregnancy termination.

At this time, only Tay-Sachs disease meets all these criteria, although sickle cell anemia is close to reaching the same point. The prenatal diagnosis of sickle cell anemia has been made, but the technique of obtaining fetal blood is yet to be evaluated for its safety and reliability.

Screening a population for carriers makes a lot of sense. The goal is to prevent the occurrence of serious hereditary disorders by providing individuals in their reproductive period with as many options as possible. They may, for example, be influenced in the choice of a mate, elect to have no children, have artificial insemination by donor, plan on adoption, or the man may opt to have a vasectomy, or the woman may have her tubes ligated. Still others may decide to have their own children, reassured by the availability of prenatal diagnosis. Certainly it is of the greatest importance to you to determine before you start to have children whether or not you are a carrier of a disorder that can be diagnosed in the fetus in early pregnancy. It is obviously too late for this approach when you've already had a child with a genetic defect. Moreover, the time for testing is *not* halfway through pregnancy. In my first book, *The Prenatal Diagnosis of Hereditary*

Disorders, written for physicians, in 1973, I suggested that the ideal time for a couple to determine whether they are carriers of certain harmful genes is when they apply for their marriage license, or at least at the time of marriage. More recently, the Chicago Bar Association echoed those sentiments and agreed with me that all couples should be offered genetic counseling and/or tests to determine if they are carriers of certain hereditary disorders that may be prevalent in their families. Only in this way can couples be certain of being spared the tragedy of having deformed or defective children. Currently the law simply requires a blood test for venereal disease!

During some of these screening programs, a number of unforeseen hazards were encountered. In the sickle cell anemia testing program for carriers, variations of that disease were detected and made for some confusion in those screened. Because many of the programs were begun in such haste and without careful preparation, a number of mistakes were made. One of the most critical problems that arose was the confusion engendered in those who were screened. Many carriers, for example, thought they themselves had the disease and thus needed special dietary or other care. This of course was incorrect. Equally disturbing was what happened during a similar type of screening program in Greece, where young women discovered to be carriers found themselves ineligible for their prearranged marriages. In the United States some carriers of sickle cell anemia were unreasonably asked to pay higher insurance premiums and were even excluded from some branches of the armed forces. Finally, since both parents are carriers of sickle cell anemia when an affected child is born, the screening program deeply embarrassed couples when it turned out that the father was in fact not a carrier. The unmasking of infidelity on the part of the mother naturally caused grave problems in a family already struck with the tragedy of a defective child.

Screening and the Future

The future of screening seems clear. Patients and physicians alike will continue to seek and determine inborn weaknesses, predispositions, or susceptibilities. Screening for hereditary diseases will be seen as a very significant effort in the prevention of disease, and the number of genetic diseases that can be diagnosed accurately, as well as the number of disorders in which the carrier state can be determined, will continue to increase steadily. It is not even too difficult to imagine that a time could come when each of us has a genetic identity card. Such a card would assist us not only in the selection of mates and in the prevention of genetic disease, but also in the treatment of diseases that we may be susceptible to at any point in our lifetime.

But first we need drastic changes in the way we think about disease. To seek medical attention only when one is sick is a hazardous way of life. It is especially hard to convince young adults of the time-honored adage: "An ounce of prevention is worth a pound of cure." In the case of hereditary disease, ten dollars' worth of prevention should be measured against a lifetime of sorrow, thousands of dollars for alleviation, and no real cure.

Though screening millions of people for genetic disorders is now a possibility, it will take a change in the public's attitude to achieve large-scale efforts. It is crucial for you to research through your family and recognize your own genetic susceptibilities.

Drugs and Other Perils

Each time you take a drug — even an aspirin — you consider the dosage and are at least aware of possible side effects. Thinking back, however, have you ever thought that you might have an inborn adverse reaction to that particular drug? Has it ever crossed your mind that a dosage of some other drug may be too much or too little for you because of your unique biochemical make-up? Some people who have seizures may need much more antiseizure medication than others because of the different ways drugs are bound and transported by blood proteins. These differences are inherited. Similarly, an individual may have a violent reaction to a single injection of penicillin that could be fatal. Again, this reaction or ana- phylaxis probably is related to the transmission through the family of an inherited allergic predisposition.

Inborn Mechanisms

As we all differ in appearance and personality, so do basic chemicals in the body differ slightly from one person to the next. These biochemical differences are important to under- stand since every individual body handles drugs in a unique way. Professor Burt N. LaDu of the New York University School of Medicine describes this as our "pharmacological individuality." The evidence is clear that this is a reflection of hereditary variability. As an example, many drugs we take have to be processed through the bowel and via the liver into the bloodstream. The drug has to be broken down by chemi- cal reactions in the body and it may have to be transferred around the body via a particular protein to which it may be hooked in various ways. The drug, or the products resulting from its breakdown, has then to pass through the cell wall to get into the cell where it can have its effect. The actual se- quence of events is even more complicated than the simplified description I have just given, but it should be sufficiently clear that heredity makes a difference in the handling of a drug by the body at each step. Inherited deficiencies of those enzymes necessary to break down a drug or to help in its excretion by the body may lead to accumulation of the drug and finally to toxic effects on the heart, the eye, the liver, and so on. Alter- natively, because of a unique, inherited system in a particular person, drugs may be so rapidly broken down by a person with a different genetic make-up that the usual dosages of drugs taken have little or no effect. In fact, about half the population of the United States and Canada breaks down isoni- azid (used in treatment of tuberculosis) slowly. In contrast, only 5 percent of Canadian Eskimos do so, while 83 percent of the Egyptians are able to break it down this way. The impli- cation again is that if a person breaks down a drug such as isoniazid slowly, much more is given than is necessary, and it may rapidly accumulate and cause such complications as nerve damage.

A Little Is Too Much

Quite a number of other drugs, including phenobarbital, are handled differently by different individuals. A potentially catastrophic situation may arise in a person who lacks an enzyme whose "job" it is to take care of particular drugs. The two most important are succinylcholine and suxamethonium, which are usually given as muscle relaxants as part of general anesthesia. The "sensitive," susceptible individual, unable to break down a drug efficiently, accumulates high concentrations of the drug in the bloodstream. Such an individual may suffer from prolonged paralysis following anesthesia and die if the situation goes unrecognized. The sensitivity to these drugs is inherited equally from parents who are both carriers. Those who carry this predisposition do not themselves show any abnormal sensitivity to these drugs. The situation is, however, not rare since about 1 in 2000 individuals and about 2 out of every 100 whites might carry this disorder! Curiously, Alaskan Eskimos have a remarkably high incidence of this sensitivity.

A Lot Is Too Little

The opposite situation has also been noted. In other words, an individual may have a much more efficient mechanism to break down the drug, and therefore may need for example almost three times more succinylcholine to achieve the same degree of relaxation under anesthesia as does a normal individual. Also, a number of persons have been identified for whom the dose of an anticoagulant drug necessary to achieve its action was about 25 times more than that expected for a normal individual. This resistance to an anticoagulant was shown to be clearly inherited.

Combinations May Be Hazardous

I am sure you are already aware that one drug may interfere with another drug taken simultaneously. For example, a patient taking isoniazid for the treatment of tuberculosis may also be taking Dilantin for epilepsy. In such a situation, the isoniazid may interfere with the handling of Dilantin, which could then accumulate in the body, yielding toxic concentrations. Such a consequence would then lead to the complications of Dilantin toxicity including jerky eye movements, loss of balance and unsteadiness in walking, drowsiness, and so on. Some of the drug-to-drug interactions probably result from inherited biochemical mechanisms.

Hereditary Disorders Associated with Adverse Drug Reactions

There are many people in all countries born with a hereditary condition that by itself causes few if any problems. However, in some of these disorders exposure to specific drugs may lead to serious complications. A large number of blacks and Orientals may have an inherited deficiency of a particular enzyme within the red blood cell, called glucose-6-phosphate dehydrogenase deficiency. If they take sulfa drugs, drugs to reduce fever, certain antimalarial drugs, and a host of others including aspirin, they may develop a hemolytic anemia (see also Chapter 6, Table 2). Between 5 to 40 percent of Italians, Greeks, and other Mediterranean and Middle Eastern peoples also have glucose-6-phosphate dehydrogenase deficiency. The defect is especially important in Greeks and Chinese, since it is commonly associated with serious jaundice in the newborn, which if not promptly treated may cause brain damage. Another complication occurs when the fetus has glucose-6-phosphate dehydrogenase deficiency and the mother takes certain medications, for example, sulfa drugs. The drugs cross over into the susceptible fetus and may cause severe anemia and even fetal death.

A person born with a variation in one of the proteins, hemoglobin, in the red blood cells may also suffer from anemia following the taking of similar drugs.

A whole host of other hereditary disorders are known that may cause particular drugs to produce unusual or even undesirable effects. Patients with inherited glaucoma, high pressure in the eye, develop even higher pressures within the eye if they are inadvertently given atropine or other drugs to dilate the pupils, and the condition may also be aggravated by some types of cortisone. Hence, it is important to find out through a simple test used by all reputable eye specialists whether you have glaucoma or not.

Patients with Down's syndrome are known to be extremely sensitive to atropine. This drug, usually given immediately prior to an operation, may even be fatal in these patients. Patients with familial dysautonomia, a disorder of the involuntary nervous system that controls blushing, blood pressure, and so on, may show a marked increase in blood pressure when given the drug noradrenalin. It also appears that some of the symptoms can be temporarily relieved by treatment with another drug called urecholine.

One day in 1932, a scientist complained that the powder his colleague was working with in the same room caused a very bitter taste. The substance, called phenylthiourea (or phenylthiocarbamide [PTC]), did not taste bitter to the man actually handling it. Quite by accident, these two had stumbled on what is now well recognized: some people are born with the inability to taste PTC. Their inability to taste PTC is inherited as a recessive gene from both parents, while the capacity to taste this bitter compound is transmitted from one parent to half the children.

The curious thing about nontasters is that they have a much higher frequency of lumps or tumors of the thyroid gland. Tasters, in contrast, more often develop overacting thyroid glands or hyperthyroidism.

There seems to be no end to the remarkable diversity of the genetic mechanisms of disorders that plague us. Consider yet another typical story of an incredible hereditary disorder:

*J.L. was twenty-two years of age, and decided that she had
had enough of recurrent severe tonsillitis and ear infections.
Her physician in desperation had recommended a tonsillec-
tomy, and she finally decided to proceed.*

*During the operation her temperature suddenly skyrocketed
to 108°F, her pulse raced at 200 per minute, and her heartbeat became grossly irregular. Her body developed extreme
muscular rigidity; she became as stiff as a board. Her quick-
thinking and alert anesthetist knew immediately what to do
(stop the anesthesia, give oxygen, force respiration, cool body
rapidly with ice, treat biochemical consequences, and so on).*

*J.L. survived unharmed, but nowadays still about 60 per-
cent of individuals die in this situation.*

Her inherited defect is called malignant hyperthermia, and
it can cause a variety of anesthetic agents to precipitate catas-
trophe. Tragedy may strike during the first, second, or subsequent operations under anesthesia. About two-thirds of the
victims are affected during their first experience with general
anesthesia. Such individuals may appear to be perfectly
healthy, but a very careful examination may reveal one or
more of the following features: droopy eyelids, crossed eyes,
curvature of the spine, double-jointedness, larger muscle bulk
(although the patient may complain of muscle weakness or
cramps), and difficulties with temperature control. Thus far,
most people never knew they had malignant hyperthermia until it occurred, and this lack of awareness often killed them.
The triggering factor appears to be general anesthesia, during
which the patient develops sudden and tremendously high
temperatures. One woman is known to have reached a temperature of 112°F and survived without apparent brain damage
— probably a world record.

Hyperthermia is transmitted as a dominant trait, so an affected parent takes a 50 percent risk in each pregnancy of
passing it on. There are so few clues on physical examination
that the first identification of the disorder may be during operation under general anesthesia. And that may be too late! It
is possible, and very important, to test anyone with a family

history of hyperthermia. Muscle biopsy enables a diagnosis to be made before an operation in about half the cases. Electrical studies of muscles, called electromyograms, show a typical pattern in about half the cases. Probably the best test at the present time is to place a tiny piece of muscle in a solution and add caffeine. Muscle from the affected person contracts more rapidly than muscle tissue of someone without hyperthermia.

Counterparts of many human diseases have been found in a variety of different animals, including cats, dogs, cows, pigs, mice, and hamsters. This provides opportunities to study the particular disease in a model system, and recent observations have shown that the pig can have a disease similar to malignant hyperthermia. Not only are these animal models extremely valuable in research for discovering the basic mechanisms of a human disease, but they also provide opportunities to try out different kinds of treatment. Consequently, for malignant hyperthermia, evidence is accumulating that the local anesthetic procaine, which works for pigs, may be valuable in the treatment of human beings.

Helpful Considerations If You Have a Hereditary Disorder

While it is not possible to cure an inborn hereditary disorder, it is possible to do a number of constructive things. Specific treatments are available that may allow one to live without undue pain, discomfort, or even ill health. The kinds of treatment available for hereditary diseases are discussed in some detail in Chapter 21. But one really cannot emphasize enough the need to be continually on the lookout for the specific complications associated with a hereditary disorder you may have.

Being aware is one thing; anticipating and preventing harm is another. A person who suffers, for instance, from the dominant hereditary disorder called pheochromocytoma, which is characterized by tumors occurring along the autonomic nervous system, has a high risk of developing cancer of the thyroid gland. Here watchfulness is all important. Blood pressure checks, examination of the thyroid gland, and blood and urine tests would all help to anticipate possible complications and catch them in time to prevent a serious outcome. In another rare condition characterized by rickets (called Vitamin D Resistant Rickets), the disease is transmitted mainly from affected males to all female offspring. Recognition of this disorder and knowledge of the mode of transmission will make it possible to insist that all daughters are given high doses of vitamin D plus additional phosphorus in the diet. If a female transmits the disease, then half the sons and half the daughters will require the same treatment.

Another example is that of polycystic kidney disease, which an affected parent will pass along to half of his or her children. Since high blood pressure is a serious hazard here, it is important to recognize one special condition that is being associated rather frequently with polycystic kidney disease. It is a small bulge in the wall of a blood vessel inside the skull (called a berry aneurysm) that can burst when the blood pressure goes too high. Hypertension in this situation can therefore not be ignored, and kidney transplantation may have to be considered.

Hereditary disorders may not be fatal, though some of their complications may cause eventual death. It is therefore vital for the affected person to remain very alert about the possibilities. Take, for example, the condition called familial polyposis of the colon. In this condition, large numbers of polyps occur in the colon and are often premalignant. Hence, whenever these polyps are found they should be surgically removed. Such an affected person is advised to have a sigmoidoscopy (examination of the colon under direct vision through a tube passed through the rectum) at least once or twice a year for life. Some have even chosen surgical removal of the entire colon to prevent any such further possible complication.

In the case of the more common ailment of sugar diabetes or diabetes mellitus, many physicians feel that all close relatives of diabetics should be tested for it once a year. It is recommended, too, that first degree relatives of those afflicted by glaucoma, also a hereditary condition, should have yearly examinations.

There are a number of other diseases in this category with long names, which would not be meaningful unless you yourself had one of them. The point really is that you should know what you have and should be aware of what possible complications may ensue. Anticipatory intervention or early diagnosis may save your life, or the life of your loved ones. Therefore, consult your doctor and explore these possibilities with this approach in mind.

To sum up:

You may get to know which harmful genes you carry if you

1. Yourself have a genetic disorder
2. Have a child with a specific hereditary disease
3. Had yourself tested because of a family history of a particular disorder
4. Are *automatically* a carrier, for instance, the daughter of a father with hemophilia
5. Had yourself tested because you belong to a certain ethnic group, such as blacks of African origin or Jews of Ashkenazic origin.

Ultimately, screening of large segments of the population may become more widespread as further research leads to progress in medical knowledge and technology. Meanwhile, if you find yourself identifying with any of the five groups just described or have concerns about symptoms we have discussed, then I advise you to consult your doctor. If the answers provided leave you uncertain, then a consultation should be sought with a medical geneticist in a large medical center associated with a medical school.

My ardent hope is that you will consider your genetic status and that of your mate before you marry, before you have children. You owe it to yourself and to your children at least to have proceeded with the best available knowledge of your genetic endowment. You have a right to know, in fact, a distinct personal obligation to know.

CHAPTER 8

Superstition and Birth Defects

THROUGHOUT THE AGES men and women have reacted to the birth of malformed offspring with awe, fear, admiration, or with a foreboding of evil and imminent disaster. Artifacts depicting remarkable malformations such as double-headed single-bodied "monsters" or other species of conjoined twins occasionally served as prototypes of gods or demigods with magic powers. It seems that in very ancient times, grossly deformed infants were regarded as divine and probably worshipped. Our fascination with major birth defects has been expressed in art for thousands of years. A sculpture of a double-headed twin goddess was discovered in southern Turkey dating back to approximately 6500 B.C.E. Chalk and wooden carvings dating back to stone-age civilizations bear witness to the powers of observation and eye for detail expressed in specimens with "Siamese-type twins," too many fingers on one hand, and so on.

During the Babylonian dynasty some 4000 years ago, congenital malformations were viewed as omens, important in foretelling the future. To quote a few Babylonian diviners, as described by J. W. Ballantyne, in 1894, in "The Teratological Records of Chaldea":

When a woman gives birth to an infant whose nostrils are absent, the country will be in affliction, and the house of the man will be ruined. When a woman gives birth to an infant that has no nose, affliction will seize upon the country, and the master of the house will die. When a woman gives birth to an infant that has no penis, the master of the house will be enriched by the harvest of his fields. When a woman gives birth to an infant that has no clear marked sex, calamity and *affliction will seize upon the land: the master of the house shall have no happiness.*

Even multiple births were regarded both in Babylonian and Roman times as portents: a food shortage was supposed to follow the birth of quadruplets. The birth of a hermaphrodite was believed to be an ill omen by the Romans and such bisexual children were executed.

The idea that the births of extremely deformed children predicted disaster remained in vogue till the close of the seventeenth century. Paradoxically, these gross-looking individuals were patronized rather than shunned and even received in the courts of Europe.

From time immemorial, some men and women have believed that a major birth defect was God's punishment for sins committed or a sign of punishment to come. It is not unusual, even today, to encounter parents who confide their innermost belief that God is punishing them for acts or sins they have committed. Some years ago, during a consultation with a mother who had brought her hydrocephalic child for evaluation, she asked if I thought it was possible that God had punished her with this second deformed child because her first, a normal child, had been run over by an automobile. The combination of her two tragedies led to her total nervous breakdown and institutionalization for many years.

One common belief is that a shock or stress or excessive worry may produce birth defects in the child. No solid evidence has accumulated to confirm any such view. During the Second World War, the bombing of London and other major English cities did not lead to an increase in the frequency of birth defects, despite overwhelming stress.

It's in the Mind

Another age-old idea, that the thoughts of the pregnant mother may affect the development of the fetus, has also not been substantiated. The power of these mental impressions, as they are called, was believed to act from the moment of conception. Children conceived out of wedlock, allegedly in great passion, were thought to be artistically gifted. Many centuries ago in Greece, expectant mothers were encouraged to look at beautiful statues and pictures in order to make their children strong and beautiful, and indeed the Spartans made laws to that effect. An old Norwegian law prohibited butchers from hanging their hares in public, because of the fear that such a sight would cause pregnant women to have children with harelip or cleft lip. Mothers have also blamed their own thoughts, moods, and emotions during pregnancy. Because certain defective infants resembled monkeys (for example, microcephalic or anencephalic babies) the view took root that it might be dangerous for pregnant women to look at monkeys. One close relative of mine elaborated on the cause of a hairy "nevus," or dark hairy birthmark. She was convinced that a sudden scare by a hairy animal (e.g., cat or mouse), during which shock the pregnant mother suddenly touched her protruding stomach, was the real cause of the birthmark. Coincidence may of course have given occasional support to such beliefs. Professor Josef Warkany, of Cincinnati, Ohio, who has spent a lifetime in the study of congenital malformations, quotes in one of his scholarly texts, *Congenital Malformations*, the following remarkable case:

A noble but curious lady attended an execution while she was pregnant. The executioner cut off one of the condemned man's hands before proceeding to his main task, the separation of the head from the body. After that hand was cut off, the lady became extremely excited, began to tremble and left hastily. Several days later she gave birth to a child who had only one hand. The severed hand was "born" some time later.

Today we recognize that intrauterine amputations of fingers or hands or even arms may occur because of the presence of severely constricting amniotic membrane bands. By coincidence, the hand of the child of the noble but curious lady was

separated in the same place where the executioner's axe fell.
(In any event, for general health reasons one might suggest
that pregnant women avoid the indulgence of watching
executions!)

Perhaps the earliest recording of the theory on prenatal reaction to outside impressions is in the Book of Genesis. Jacob,
having been promised by his father-in-law that he would be
left all the mottled and speckled lambs and kids, secured his
inheritance by placing partly peeled, streaked, and mottled
branches of trees in the area where the animals conceived. He
then mingled the offspring conceived under these circum-
stances among the flocks, and further increased the number of
spotted, speckled, and streaked animals. He was, possibly,
simply a brilliant geneticist?

So-called irrational beliefs or ideas of the past should not
be discarded without at least some consideration. For example, a sudden shock *could* release the adrenal hormone cortisone, which has been proved to cause cleft palate in some
strains of mice. Also, chickens exposed to excessive noise
have produced offspring with a higher frequency of birth defects. Whether the mechanism is through the release of cortisone because of stress or some other metabolic pathway is
unknown. Needless to say, one cannot and should not extrapolate too literally from the animal to the human condition, in
spite of our tendency to do so.

Between Man and Animal

Breeding between species of mammals is well known, a good
example being the horse and the donkey: the resulting mules
are particularly valuable because of their hardiness. While no
offspring can result from human and animal hybridization, in
ancient times a belief was prevalent, probably originating
from Egypt and India, that different species can fertilize each
other and thereby produce monstrous offspring, and the idea
of a cross between human and animal was not considered re-
pulsive. If a woman gave birth to a grossly malformed child
who resembled a particular animal, that child was given the

same respect that that animal enjoyed according to the official religion of the time. Professor Warkany relates that the Egyptian mummy of a human anencephalic infant was discovered in a grave apparently reserved for sacred animals. The speculation is that this grossly malformed infant appeared to resemble a monkey, and was therefore embalmed and buried with other sacred creatures. In those days, "monstrous" babies were apparently not considered unnatural, not necessarily stemming from sinful intercourse, and did not lead to the persecution of the mother. Greek mythology is replete with descriptions of centaurs (half-human–half-horse), the Minotaur (half-man–half-bull) and satyrs (goatlike creatures).

All of these pagan ideas were condemned at the time by the Christian laws that made relations between humans and animals a criminal act. In the wake of the appearance of such laws, the birth of a monstrous offspring occasionally placed both mother and father in a dangerous situation.

An example of Protestant paganism in our own country is documented in the records of the colony and plantation of New Haven (1638–1649) and is described by Professor Warkany:

It eventuated that some years after the founding of this colony, a pig was born with a major malformation involving the face and head. There was only one eye in the middle of the face and a flesh-like hollow projection in place of a nose. This particular malformation is not unusual in that species, and indeed the malformation of cyclopia (only one eye present) with a proboscis-like organ in the middle of the face instead of the nose does also (though rarely) occur in human malformed infants. As the record showed, the people at that time attributed the birth of this "monster" to the "unnatureall spell and abominable filthynes" of a servant, George Spencer, who they said had "butt one eye for use, the other hath (as itt is called) a pearle in itt" — which closely resembled the eye of the deformed pig.

Believe it or not, George Spencer was hauled into court for a trial that lasted from 1641 to 1642. The confessions and retractions as well as the testimonies have been recorded in great detail. George Spencer was found guilty and executed on April 8, 1642!

Heaven knows how many victims met their death that way. Certainly punishment was not rare. The Danish anatomist Bartholin described a girl who gave birth to a "monster" with "a cat's head" and was burned alive in the public square of Copenhagen in 1683.

Satan

The devil, witches, sorcerers, and other demonic creatures occupied the imagination of people during the fifteenth and sixteenth centuries. Birth defects such as club feet or hairy birthmarks were interpreted as signs of the devil. Occasionally mothers of such offspring were punished if not killed. In many cultures, deformed children were quickly disposed of. The Greeks and Romans practiced infanticide not only on deformed children, but on normal offspring when economic or religious considerations so demanded; even Plato advocated it for the "inferior" or deformed offspring. In Sparta, infanticide was incorporated into the constitution and practiced for the good of the commonwealth!

A belief in the evil eye originated before the beginning of recorded history. The ancient Greek philosophers taught that visual rays were emitted by the eyes. These rays were reflected back from the object to the eye. Pregnant women were therefore cautioned to be wary; exposure to the evil eye might cause the birth of a defective child.

The Horoscope

As far back as 2800 B.C.E. the Chaldean astrologers connected the occurrence of birth defects with the movements or relative positions of the planets. From time to time eclipses were claimed to cause defects, as evidenced in Sicily during the sixteenth century. Even today, there are strong believers in astrological forecasts.

Despite our collective worldliness and life-styles ruled by science, we still know little about the exact cause of many different birth defects. Hysteria and fear, born of ignorance, can easily still make inroads into our thoughts. The philosopher Spinoza concluded that superstition was engendered, preserved, and fostered by fear. Thus, it is not at all unlikely that until we have a very clear understanding of the causes of all birth defects, superstition founded on fear will continue unabated.

CHAPTER 9

Hereditary Birth Defects and Mental Retardation

A BIRTH DEFECT GENERALLY implies that a child has been born with some kind of physical sign that is abnormal, though invisible biochemical disorders are also correctly dubbed as "birth defects." The obvious congenital (born with) defects may vary in intensity from a single birthmark on the skin to a hole-in-the-heart, to grotesque facial abnormalities or even two-headed "monsters." These defects, as well as mental retardation, *may* be due to hereditary factors, even in the absence of a family history. On the other hand, they may occur together or separately due to known factors that affected the fetus during development in the womb, but were *not* hereditary and, as mentioned earlier, are known as acquired birth defects.

It may not be possible to discover the cause of either a specific birth defect or of mental retardation. The failure to find a cause for mental retardation may occur as often as in 30 to 40 percent of cases. Difficulty may also be experienced in distinguishing hereditary from acquired causes, as in cleft lip and palate, which are most often hereditary, but may also be caused by drugs taken by the pregnant woman.

Very careful analysis of the family history may point to a particular genetic disease. Photographs of affected family members living elsewhere may lead to recognition of an unusual disorder. Hospital records and autopsy reports on a previously affected child or relative are again of the greatest importance in diagnosis. Finally, actual physical examination of the parents of an affected child may provide some diagnostic leads. Such a scrutiny of the parents may even include x-rays of the skull. Tuberous sclerosis, as we saw in Chapter 7, may be inherited directly from one parent who looks entirely normal, though x-rays may reveal characteristic deposits of calcium in the brain, implying that that parent actually has the disease but shows no outward manifestations.

Obviously every effort should be made to find out the cause of a birth defect or mental retardation, since recognition of the cause is really the primary step to prevention of its recurrence.

How Frequent?

Professor Paul Polani at Guy's Hospital in London estimated that 6 percent or more of all persons "suffer from developmental disorders manifest at birth or in early life ranging from mild to severe, from curable through irremediable to untreatable or even lethal." Certainly *major* birth defects with or without serious mental retardation occur in 3 to 4 percent of all births. In the United States alone, estimates suggest that each year about 100,000 babies are born with serious birth defects and/or mental retardation. On a cumulative basis, this implies that there are approximately 6 million individuals in our country who are mentally retarded! This is a very serious public health concern.

As we mentioned earlier, in the United States and other Western countries 25 to 30 percent of all major children's hospital admissions stem from birth defects, genetic disease, or mental retardation. Minor birth defects occur in between 6 and 14 percent of all births. These and other minor signs can generally be ignored per se, though care has to be taken at first that they do not signal the presence of something more serious, such as a heart or brain defect.

Gross birth defects are a different matter, and are responsible for about 15 percent of deaths in the newborn period.

Causes

Abnormalities of the Chromosomes

We discussed (in Chapters 2 and 3) how a person may be born with too many chromosomes, too few chromosomes, or abnormalities in the structure of particular chromosomes. About 1 in 200 children is born with chromosome abnormalities that may or may not be associated with mental retardation.

In the United States alone, each year close to 20,000 children are born with chromosomal abnormalities. At least one-half of these involve the parents as well as the child. Confronted by a child with an unusual appearance or mental retardation, it is a relatively simple matter to obtain a blood sample to document the normality or abnormality of the chromosomes. The commonest disorder in this group of conditions is of course Down's syndrome.

Birth Defects Transmitted from One Parent

There are many different recognized birth defects that can be transmitted from one affected parent, each child having a 50 percent chance of being affected or suffering from dominant inheritance. Some of these disorders are minor and include conditions such as incurved fifth fingers or extra digits. Some are more severe, as when one parent has a hand or hands resembling a lobster claw. As shown in Chapter 5, each new pregnancy in that family carries a 50 percent risk that the offspring will have a similar deformity.

A parent may have markedly underdeveloped cheekbones (maxillas), but no other defects. An affected child (the risk being 50 percent) may be born missing an ear, and the underdeveloped cheekbones may also affect the shape and appearance of the eyes, and these defects form the Treacher-Collins syndrome.

A white forelock of hair in a parent may signal that half the children may be born deaf, or have disabilities of less consequence. The disorder is known as Waardenburg's syndrome.

Extra digits or polydactyly is seen in infants quite frequently. Close to 1 in every 100 black newborns has an extra finger and/or toe on one or both feet. Polydactyly may also be simply inherited from one parent as dominant inheritance. Occasionally, parents will vehemently deny any family history of this minor defect. On being asked to look at their hands, some of them find a tiny scar at the base of their fifth fingers, which they had not known about. The scar indicates the site of the extra tiny finger that had simply been tied off at birth, which then fell off shortly thereafter.

Hernias of the navel (umbilicus) and a tiny hole in front of the ears called a preauricular fistula are other harmless birth defects that are especially common in blacks. Both disappear without any treatment or surgery.

Much has been written about birth defects as related to the increasing age of the mother (see Chapter 15). There are, however, a few defects — albeit rare — that are associated with the increased age of the father. Achondroplasia is one example of such a defect. The father is frequently over forty or fifty years old, but is seemingly normal. There are some other conditions, a few involving bones, muscles, connective tissues or joints, called Marfan's syndrome, Apert's syndrome, and myositis ossificans progressiva, where the correlation with older fathers is suspected but not as well established. One other rare disorder in this group is a defect or absence of the iris (the colored part of the eye), which may signal a tumor of the kidney. Yearly or twice yearly physical examinations of the child are necessary to ensure that no genetically predisposed defect, for example, cancer of the kidney, develops without being recognized in time.

Birth Defects When Both Parents Are Normal but Are Carriers

Most of the disorders found in this category involve biochemical disturbances in the child leading usually to mental retardation, but without deformation of the limbs or face. Many of these biochemical disorders of metabolism are diagnosable prenatally, and the chance that they may occur in each pregnancy is 25 percent (for example, Tay-Sachs disease or Gaucher's disease). We mentioned earlier birth defects and mental retardation resulting from the marriage of close relatives or as a consequence of incest (see Chapter 6).

Sometimes disorders in this group cause visible physical abnormalities, as in certain types of microcephaly or small headedness, which imply mental retardation. A number of birth defects occurring consistently together are referred to as a syndrome. Some of these syndromes may be transmitted from both parents as recessive inheritance, neither of them being affected themselves. In each pregnancy the risk of recurrence is 25 percent. The otopalato-digital syndrome is one example, the affected child having a face with unusual features of eyebrows and nose, a "long" head, cleft palate, markedly enlarged tips of fingers and toes, extremely short big toes, and slow physical and mental development. One particularly important disorder in this group may be confused with serious defects of the brain, such as anencephaly, or spinal cord disease, such as spina bifida, discussed in detail below. Recognition of this condition, called Meckel's syndrome, invariably associated with fatal malformations of the brain, extra digits, and kidney abnormalities is very important because the risk of recurrence in each pregnancy is 25 percent, as opposed to the 3 to 5 percent for the anencephaly group.

Birth Defects with Mother as Carrier and Only Sons Affected

It has been known for about 40 years that an excess of males with mental retardation are found both in institutions for the mentally retarded and the general population. This is most pronounced among those who are severely retarded. While it is also known that, for some strange reasons, males more often suffer birth injury, this is not sufficient reason to account for the disparity between the sexes in subsequent mental retardation. Careful studies of the family histories in some of these cases have drawn attention to the fact that at least in some instances the mother is the carrier. Such mothers have a 50 percent chance that each of their sons could have mental retardation. Usually there is no other associated birth defect. Nor is it possible to detect the carrier mother. One case I vividly recall illustrates the point well.

I saw Mr. and Mrs. C in consultation with their two sons, aged four and eight. Both boys were moderately retarded and no cause had been found by the referring doctor. Mrs. C's pregnancy had been perfectly normal. She had had no infections, no fevers, taken no drugs, and suffered no injuries. Both she and her husband were perfectly normal.

Physical examination of both boys showed no abnormalities other than the mental retardation. Futhermore, a whole battery of special tests to try and determine the cause of their mental retardation were all unproductive.

The answer lay in their family history. On Mr. C's side of the family, there were no instances of mental retardation, birth defects, or genetic disease. However, Mrs. C had one brother who was mentally retarded (from no known cause) and four sisters. Two of the sisters had each had one son with mental retardation, the third sister had had three sons afflicted with it. The fourth sister was unmarried. Looking further back into Mrs. C's family, on her mother's side there were two uncles who were retarded as well. No retarded females were noted in the entire family pedigree.

This was a clear case of a sex-linked disorder: retardation affecting half the males born to a female carrier. The family was reassured that they could safely have girls. This they did by utilizing prenatal diagnosis, and achieved the birth of two girls in consecutive pregnancies — something they might not have done without the reassurance provided by prenatal diagnosis.

Some experts have calculated that as many as 20 percent of severely mentally retarded boys (I.Q.'s less than 50) may be the victims of this sex-linked inheritance. Clearly, therefore, careful analysis of the family history is crucial in these cases since prenatal sex determination is now possible, and parents may avoid the risk by choosing to have girls.

Many birth defects, with or without mental retardation, are transmitted by the mother in the same way. Types of hydrocephalus (large heads with increased fluid in the brain and often associated with mental retardation), a failure of the intestine to open at the anus (imperforate anus), small deformed blind eyes (microphthalmia), and certain other biochemical disorders of metabolism are but a few examples.

Birth Defects with Parents Usually Unaffected and with Operating Environmental and Genetic Factors

This form of multifactorial or polygenic inheritance reflects the combined effects of several minor gene abnormalities acting in concert with environmental factors. Two of the most serious occur most commonly in children of Irish ancestry. The brain defect called anencephaly is incompatible with life, while children with a spinal defect, spina bifida, may have major health problems and a markedly decreased life expectancy. A child affected with anencephaly is likely to be stillborn or dies within minutes to hours of birth, or sometimes lingers on even for two or three months before dying. The spinal defect, in contrast, is not fatal, but repairing the open spine usually results in paralysis of the legs (paraplegia) and frequently lack of control of bowel and bladder functions. The child may be mentally normal, but confined to a wheel chair and may leak urine, sometimes stool, constantly. The effect on the child and family can well be imagined. Occasionally, the spinal lesion is sufficiently small to be repaired without any disability remaining, the person being able to walk and function normally. (For prenatal diagnosis of these defects see Chapter 16.)

Environmental factors seem especially strong in the cases of both anencephaly and spina bifida. As we mentioned before, in Northern Ireland, the frequency of these conditions is about 7 in every 1000 births and this high rate drops gradually as one moves to the south of England where the frequency is about 2 to 3 per 1000 births. Strange as it seems, and totally unexplained, these anencephaly and spina bifida conditions occur with the same high frequency in northern India, and Alexandria, Egypt, as in Northern Ireland. Besides geographical effects, there are recognizable seasonal effects, in that more frequent winter and fall births have often been observed. Finally some relationship between poverty as well as illegitimacy has been shown for these defects.

There are other birth defects besides the anencephaly/spina

bifida group that are caused by the interaction of genetic and environmental factors. These include cleft lip and/or palate, club feet, pyloric stenosis, which is a congenital block at the exit of the stomach into the intestine, dislocated hips, certain congenital heart defects (e.g., atrial septal defect) to mention only the most common physically obvious defects.

Professor Cedric O. Carter at the Hospital for Sick Children, Great Ormond Street, London, has studied how frequently these defects recur in families. Since these conditions are quite common, it might be helpful if I gave some guiding figures for most of the disorders mentioned.

For the nervous system disorders, note that parents may have a child with anencephaly and later in another pregnancy have a child with spina bifida.

For all the defects mentioned above:

If one parent is affected	the risk of having an affected child is about 3–5%.
If the parents are normal and they have had one affected child	the risk of having another is about 3–5%.
If the parents are normal and they have had 2 affected children	the risk is about 8–12% for having a third affected child.
If normal parents have had 3 affected children	the risk is about 25% for having another affected child.

The general risks for first cousins, nephews and nieces for all these disorders is thought to be higher than in the population at large. The first cousins of spina bifida patients have about an eightfold increase in risk relative to the general population.

Even for the group of disorders we are discussing, sex differences are often quite prominent. Males are much more often affected by pyloric stenosis, cleft lip and/or palate, and club feet. In contrast, many more females are born with anencephaly and congenital dislocation of the hips.

The recurrence figures for pyloric stenosis (narrowing of duodenum) are somewhat different from the *general guidelines* expressed above.

If the mother had pyloric stenosis
>> the risk is 16–20% for having an affected son.
>> the risk is about 7% for having an affected daughter.

If the father had pyloric stenosis
>> the risk is about 5% for having an affected son.
>> the risk is about 2.5% for having an affected daughter.

For a girl with pyloric stenosis
>> any future brother has a risk of 10%.
>> any future sister has a risk of 4%.

For a boy with pyloric stenosis
>> any future brother has a risk of 4%.
>> any future sister has a risk of 2.5%.

Hereditary Disease in the Mother That May Affect the Child

A mother who herself has a genetic disease or is only a carrier may of course transmit that disorder to her children. However, besides that eventuality, her disease, genetic or otherwise, may cause problems or complications to the fetus while in the womb, or to the child when subsequently born.

The best single example (admittedly rare) is of a mother having phenylketonuria, a hereditary biochemical disorder in which the untreated patient usually has mental retardation. In such a case, the diagnosis of a biochemical disorder may never have been made, but such an affected mother who becomes pregnant damages the developing brain of the fetus. Virtually every child she brings into the world will have mental retardation, and a fair number will have additional birth defects!

Diabetes in the mother has been associated many times with an increased frequency of birth defects in the offspring (see Chapter 21). It is likely that the severity and duration of diabetes, and the various types of drugs that are used in its control, could possibly have some bearing on this. Recent evidence has indicated a significant lowering of intelligence in children of diabetic mothers, especially if the mothers had experienced episodes of poor diabetic control during pregnancy. Two quite different types of birth defects appear to be correlated with diabetes in the mother. One is a major deformity of the lower end of the spine, called caudal dysplasia, and the other is a congenital heart defect, called transposition of the great arteries, in which the major blood vessels emerging from the heart arise from the wrong heart chambers. The latter occurs 3 to 5 times more often in the babies of diabetic mothers. These children often have somewhat large, puffy, red faces, are possibly jittery, are more susceptible to respiratory distress, and have problems with low blood sugar. All these features are, however, transient. If a baby's birth weight is high (e.g., over ten pounds), it would be wise for the mother to have a glucose tolerance test for hidden (latent) diabetes.

The mother may be affected by another hereditary biochemical disorder called galactosemia that may damage the brain of the fetus and cause mental retardation. Both for phenylketonuria and galactosemia, specific diets during pregnancy may avert damage to the fetus.

Mothers with sickle cell anemia, like diabetic mothers, have a higher likelihood of losing babies around the time of delivery. In fact, 12 to 39 percent of their offspring are apt to die. An increased frequency of prematurity has also been noted, with its associated complications of respiratory distress or jaundice.

While mothers with sickle cell anemia or cystic fibrosis may not have offspring with significant abnormalities, they may themselves succumb to complications of their own disorder aggravated by pregnancy. Women with these two hereditary disorders need very good medical care and should always give serious consideration to not having children.

Mothers who have underacting thyroid glands (hypothyroidism) or overacting thyroid glands (hyperthyroidism) appear to have an increased chance of having children with chromosomal abnormalities. Reports from one large study at

Yale University School of Medicine suggested an eightfold increase for mothers with hyperthyroidism for bearing a child with chromosomal abnormalities such as Down's syndrome.

We have taken a most cursory look in this chapter at some of the hereditary types of birth defects and mental retardation. The environment provides a remarkable number of factors that may cause birth defects or mental retardation, which we should now look at most carefully.

CHAPTER 10

The Unseen Enemy: Infection and X-rays

MENTAL RETARDATION OR BIRTH DEFECTS may be caused by a variety of agents found in the environment. The important point is that, in contrast to harmful genes, they can be prevented before birth, though infection may of course occur any time after birth and lead to mental retardation. In this and the next chapter, our focus is on factors that affect the fetus in the womb, whether they be infection, x-rays, or drugs. The social and economic drain on society resulting from the care necessary for damaged and defective children is simply enormous. The German measles epidemic of 1964 cost the United States an estimated $920 million for institutional care and special educational facilities, let alone the anguish to the families involved.

Infection

Infection contracted by the mother during pregnancy is an important cause of imperfect development of the fetus. Recent estimates from major United States government studies suggest that as many as 10 percent of all cases of mental retardation may be attributed to infectious diseases. While German measles in pregnancy is well known by many people as a cause of birth defects, other infections may cause equally devastating results. One important problem is that they are often hidden and not clinically apparent. Such possibilities have worried me all too often since I know that a mother who may actually have mild German measles or another virus infection may simply feel out of sorts, have no fever, but nevertheless be in a position to infect her fetus seriously!

Timing of the Insult

The stages of development from the fertilized egg, to the embryo, to the fetus are well recognized. In the first three months, when all systems and organs are developing in the fetus, there are *critical* periods when the eyes are developing, the heart chambers are closing, the limbs are beginning to form, and so on. Sometimes, looking back, it may be possible to estimate fairly accurately at what stage in the first three months of pregnancy a particular insult or infection to the embryo occurred. The matter is complicated by the fact that viruses or drugs, acting on the developing fetus early in pregnancy, may have very different effects from case to case. Even German measles contracted during the first three months of pregnancy does not *invariably* cause birth defects.

German Measles (Rubella)

An Australian ophthalmologist first observed in 1941 that German measles during early pregnancy could cause what is now recognized to be a pattern of birth defects called the rubella syndrome. About 8 to 10 percent of all women of childbearing age today are still susceptible to German measles. In spite of immunization efforts, massive epidemics of rubella occur worldwide in cycles. During the last major one in 1964, in the United States alone over 20,000 children were born with serious birth defects.

Women exposed to rubella in early pregnancy have fetuses that show evidence of infection in up to 50 percent of cases. Some studies have shown a risk of 61 percent following exposure in the first four weeks of pregnancy, 26 percent for exposure between the fifth and eighth weeks, and 8 percent from nine to twelve weeks. The major abnormalities that occur affect the eye (cataracts), the ears (deafness), the heart ("hole-in-the-heart") and the brain (mental retardation). Other important defects include growth failure, failure to thrive, bone involvement, or skin rashes. Studies over the last few years have shown that the most common cause of deafness in a child with no other abnormalities is probably exposure of the fetus to rubella in pregnancy.

More recently it has become apparent that *even* after the first three months of pregnancy, rubella can cause mental retardation, learning disorders, deafness, and other disabilities.

Twins exposed to viral infection transmitted by the mother during pregnancy are usually both affected. However, there have been exceptions, even with German measles, where only one twin has been affected. In the case of rubella, there is another extremely important hazard to consider. The newborn baby, infected by rubella virus while a fetus in the womb, is usually still infectious and can therefore infect the people around it. Some years ago, I was called in consultation to look at a three-pound-one-ounce baby born six weeks premature who, I found, had a major heart defect. At that time, there were no other associated problems and in my consultation note I cautioned that rubella could not be excluded as the cause of the heart defect. I said it would be judicious, therefore, to isolate the baby until the diagnosis of rubella was excluded. For some reason this advice was not followed. Four weeks later I learned that one of the nurses caring for that baby had come down with German measles herself. Worse still, she was eight weeks pregnant at the time of exposure. Only after she had been diagnosed as having German measles was the child I saw tested. Sadly, but not unexpectedly, that child was found to be excreting rubella virus. The nurse and her husband decided on religious grounds not to terminate her pregnancy. They subsequently had an infant also afflicted with rubella and multiple defects.

A second case I recall was similar in that a newborn child with a group of defects suggesting rubella infection in early pregnancy was not isolated in the nursery. The child infected three members of the nursing staff, one of whom was pregnant. She delivered a blind and deaf child.

How can you prevent "silent" infection from German measles? There is only one way: be sure that the mother-to-be is immunized before pregnancy. (Some states have made rubella immunization mandatory.) The best time for rubella immunization is in the teens, or perhaps better, some months before marriage. Since live virus is used in immunization, it cannot be given during pregnancy, or for two to three months prior to conception. If rubella vaccination is given inadvertently without the woman knowing she is pregnant, then the estimated risk that the fetus will be infected is between 5 to 10 percent: a risk high enough to justify abortion. An additional safeguard is to provide a blood sample prior to pregnancy and have the serum studied (and also stored frozen) for the level of antibodies to rubella (or other viruses). If natural immunity has been established by infection years before, as reflected by a good level of antibodies, then rubella immunization is not needed. Unfortunately, women previously immunized against rubella infection may still, though rarely, have affected offspring, in contrast to those who have had a case of German measles itself. To reiterate, it is wise for all women to determine if they are susceptible to rubella and to take steps to obtain immunization *prior* to pregnancy.

Other Infections

Except for rubella and syphilis, which are both associated with birth defects, the correlation of other infectious disorders with such problems is debatable. Reports from both England and the United States have concluded that no clear causal relationship exists between birth defects and infection of the mother with chicken pox, measles, mumps, influenza, poliomyelitis, or hepatitis. Nevertheless, there are at least 13 cases described where major birth defects occurred after chicken pox during a pregnancy. Thus, no assurance can or should be given for the viral disorders mentioned above, including herpes, Coxsackie, or mononucleosis viral infections. Herpes infection — the virus that causes cold sores or blisters on the lips — may cause similar sores around or in the vagina. During birth, the baby may pick up this infection on the way out and become seriously ill, even retarded, from infection acquired in the birth canal. Most physicians would even do a cesarean section to prevent the baby from coming into contact with such infections.

Next in importance to rubella as a cause of birth defects and/ or mental retardation is infection by a large virus (cytomegalovirus). This virus may affect as many as 6 in every 100 pregnant women. The ominous aspect of this disorder is that there are usually no symptoms, or occasionally only a mild influenzalike illness. Certainly, when rubella is not epidemic, this virus is probably the most common infectious cause of mental retardation known. The consequences of infection while in the womb are similar to rubella. Mental retardation, eye defects, and infection of the heart, liver, and other organs may occur separately or together.

As in rubella, affected newborn infants may be infectious, and should be strictly isolated in the nursery. Pregnant women should of course not take care of such infected infants. Luckily a significant number of infants with cytomegalovirus simply excrete the virus and have no actual defects.

Blood tests are available to determine if a woman is susceptible to cytomegalovirus. Again, while no vaccine is yet available, a stored serum sample may be useful for comparison with a new sample should there be a suspicious infection during pregnancy, allowing the doctor to detect a brisk rise in antibody levels to that virus, which indicates an active infection. While it is apparently rare, it is possible for a woman to have a second infected child, even to have antibodies in her blood.

Another infectious agent, a protozoan called *Toxoplasma*, may also affect the fetus in pregnancy. For example, in New York, the incidence of toxoplasmosis has been estimated to be as high as 4 to 6 per 1000 pregnancies with congenital defects resulting from these cases as frequently as 1 in every 1000 births. As in the case of rubella and cytomegalovirus infection, this organism may infect the pregnant mother without causing symptoms. When symptoms do occur, they include mild fever, malaise, muscle pains, and may be associated with enlarged glands and spleen, as well as a rash. The defects in the affected child may include mental retardation and involvement of multiple organs. A French study found that approximately 16 percent of pregnant women were susceptible to infection by *Toxoplasma*. The risks observed seemed greater for younger females. It is perhaps not widely known that domestic pets such as cats and birds may harbor *Toxoplasma* infections. Unlike rubella, cytomegalovirus, syphilis, and herpes virus infections toxoplasmosis is not communicated from person to person. Obviously, therefore, women planning pregnancies are best advised to exclude such pets from their immediate environs.

It may be possible through blood tests to determine prior to pregnancy whether you have already had toxoplasmosis, cytomegalovirus, or some other infection. You may be found to be susceptible, that is, without antibodies in your blood against these infections, and unfortunately no vaccine is yet available. As I have said in connection with other infections, one solution is to store a frozen serum sample, and if an infection is suspected during early pregnancy, the sample can be thawed and tested. A high level of antibodies in the pregnancy sample compared to the original negative stored sample would imply an active recent infection and open the *option* for pregnancy termination. It is again fortunate that about 90 percent of infected pregnancies end with normal children. For toxoplasmosis, mothers with antibodies in their blood are not usually considered in any danger of having an affected child.

In an important study done in New York City, the researchers observed that more affluent white women developed toxoplasmosis in pregnancy than those in lower socioeconomic brackets. They concluded that these women had greater access to all kinds of meat and were probably eating undercooked beef or pork. Animals (whose meat we eat) become infected, just as we do, by contact with cat feces!

X-rays During Pregnancy

It has been known for some time that exposure of the fetus to x-rays can lead to serious abnormalities such as small heads (microcephaly) with associated retardation, bone defects in the skull, spinal and eye defects, cleft palate, and severe limb deformities. Any possible doubt about this was removed after the studies made on the children of Japanese women who were pregnant in Hiroshima at the time of the atomic bomb explosions. They showed a high incidence of mental retardation and microcephaly as the earliest manifestations of problems seen in those babies born alive.

The fetus can inadvertently be irradiated when the mother has x-rays (such as of the bowel, back, or kidney) without realizing that she is pregnant. The question of fetal well-being in these instances is difficult, if not impossible, to resolve. Even if genetic studies of the amniotic fluid cells show some evidence of chromosomal damage, one cannot necessarily conclude that the fetus itself has been damaged.

Usually the fetus and subsequently the child will show no signs of abnormality. However, even in the absence of demonstrable chromosomal change, the fetus may have received sufficient irradiation as to cause microcephaly, associated invariably with mental retardation, with or without multiple birth defects. Parental anxiety is thus quite justified.

Some guidance is provided by the dose of irradiation given to the mother during the first four months of pregnancy. If it was in excess of 10 rad (a measure of irradiation), then most physicians would feel that the risk of fetal damage was very high. A dose between 5 and 10 rad, however, would be considered by some to be chancy, while most will hold that exposures of under 5 rad carry no clear risk of damage. Some real dilemmas may arise, as you can see in the following story:

Elaine was twenty-five years old and four months pregnant when she came for genetic counseling. In retrospect, she believed that she must have been about three weeks pregnant when she had a series of x-rays. At that time she had been vomiting repeatedly and her doctor could not find an explanation. A pregnancy test given at that time was negative, and he therefore ordered a GI series (x-rays of stomach and small intestines), a barium enema x-ray (for large intestine), and followed that with x-rays of her gallbladder. After all these tests were completed without demonstration of any abnormality, a pregnancy test was again performed. This test was found to be positive, and it was realized that irradiation must have occurred at about three weeks of pregnancy.

Elaine and her husband requested an amniocentesis and prenatal genetic studies to determine whether the irradiation had affected the fetus. I did not recommend that an amniocentesis be done because if we found no evidence of chromosomal damage suggesting irradiation effect in the amniotic fluid cells, then we could still not say that the fetus would be unaffected. On the other hand, if we did find effects of irradiation in the amniotic fluid cells, we could still not be sure that the fetus — though clearly exposed — would ultimately be defective in any way.

Nevertheless, this couple decided to go ahead and have the amniocentesis and prenatal chromosomal analysis that did show that some 14 percent of the cells studied had, what we believed to be, the effects of either irradiation or a virus infection. In considering the possibility of an elective abortion, the couple sought other counseling opinions. The opinions all concurred and indicated that no conclusion could be made about the fetal status or well-being. Thereupon they requested and had a second amniocentesis, the results of which were similar to the first sample. They were naturally very concerned about the kinds of damage irradiation might cause, and it was explained that microcephaly, mental retardation and/or various birth defects were possible. In the face of all they had been through, the couple decided together to continue the pregnancy. Their child at birth looked perfectly normal, and blood and skin chromosomes were normal!

While infections and x-rays during pregnancy may cause birth defects and mental retardation, drugs cause, measure for measure, many more anxieties. The drug question is complex and deserves separate and detailed consideration.

CHAPTER 11

Drugs Spell Danger

YOU MAY HAVE THOUGHT that no pregnant woman need be reminded of the dangers inherent in taking drugs. The consequences may be very serious, yet, despite all that has been said and written on the subject these past few years, pregnant women still take a remarkable amount of drugs.

A study in Scotland recently revealed that the average pregnant woman takes at least four different medications during pregnancy, and some women indulge in as many as fourteen. It is difficult enough to discover what one drug may do, let alone the potential effects of two or more on the fetus.

Proving that a particular medication does or does not cause birth defects may be extremely difficult. For example, it was first shown that thalidomide did not cause defects in rats and mice even in large doses. It did, however, cause defects in man and monkeys and to a lesser degree in rabbits. It was remarkable but true that many women who took thalidomide did not have deformed babies. It has also become clear that many different agents may produce the same pattern of defects. This is best exemplified by the fact that at least 30 techniques have been established that can cause cleft lip and palate in the laboratory animal and these include usage of vitamin A, aspirin, cortisone, x-rays and even just puncturing the amniotic sac with a needle! The problem is complicated, of course, by the frequency of birth defects caused by heredity or agents of the environment other than drugs.

Aspirin

The commonly used aspirin has clearly been demonstrated to cause birth defects in rats, mice, and monkeys when administered in very high dosages. Even "normal" dosages may not be safe in pregnancy, since the observation has been made that the potential of a given dose of aspirin for causing birth defects in *rats* can appreciably be increased by concurrent administration of benzoic acid, a widely used food preservative!

Thus far, in man no clear definite relationship has been established between aspirin ingestion and subsequent birth defects, although a Finnish study did suggest a higher frequency of defective babies born to mothers who have taken aspirin during the first three months of pregnancy. In pregnant laboratory animals, aspirin ingestion has been associated with reduced fetal weight, disappearance of the embryo (reabsorption by the body), and excessive bleeding at delivery. In smaller dosages, pregnant rats given aspirin have produced offspring with impaired learning ability.

In one large Australian study published in 1975, the babies of mothers who took aspirin regularly in pregnancy were compared to those born to mothers who did not. The former were found to have a significantly reduced birth weight, an increased level of aspirin in their own blood, and an increased death rate around the time of delivery. The incidence of birth defects was *not* significantly higher in that group. The regular aspirin takers themselves had an increased incidence of anemia, more frequent vaginal bleeding both before birth and after birth, longer pregnancies, and a higher frequency of complicated deliveries. *Aspirin* or drugs *containing* aspirin are therefore best avoided in pregnancy.

Antibiotics

A number of antibiotics have been implicated through retrospective studies of women who took such medications in the first three months of pregnancy. While some of these drugs are known to cause birth defects in animals, no clear evidence is available to suggest more than a possibility for causing birth defects in man. Some tetracycline drugs taken in pregnancy may cause permanent staining of the first teeth, and even in the second teeth emerging years later.

Vitamins

It would seem to be safest for pregnant women to curtail taking any drugs during the first four months with the exception of iron and vitamins in normal dosage. There is the occasional mother who believes that taking an excessive amount of vitamins will make her baby really strong! Unfortunately, it has already clearly been shown in a number of laboratory animals that taking excessive vitamin A during pregnancy may cause a variety of birth defects. In the human, birth malformations of the urinary tract have been reported in mothers taking excess amounts of vitamin A in the first three months.

Tranquilizers

Perhaps pregnant mothers may have a tendency to believe that what is safe for them may also be safe for their embryo or fetus. The thalidomide disaster clearly exemplifies how incorrect such thinking is. This drug was recommended as a tranquilizer and antiemetic. An alert Food and Drug Administration prevented the introduction of this drug into the United States. It did, however, become very popular in West Germany and England, where disastrous and tragic consequences followed the ingestion of this drug during pregnancy. Thousands of children were born with arms and legs either absent, incredibly deformed, grossly shortened, or useless. Some of the children were found to have defects of the heart, eyes, intestine, ears, and kidneys as well.

The time the drug was taken was shown to be crucial. The dreadful deformities of the arms and legs occurred in those children whose mothers took thalidomide on the thirtieth day after conception, whereas thalidomide taken on the thirty-fifth day resulted in defects of the lower limbs only. It was also noted that the dosage was possibly of less importance than the timing, since no matter how large or small the dose of thalidomide, when it was taken on the appropriate day, the same degree of deformities resulted. Some protective mechanisms must exist, to explain why some mothers who took it at the relevant time escaped the blight of thalidomide. The effect was also noted to vary if twins were present, in that one might be more severely affected than the other, though simultaneously exposed.

Parenthetically, defects resembling thalidomide-induced malformations do occur sporadically without apparent reason, or, even more rarely, when one parent has such a defect. There is also a hereditary type of these malformations seen in the handless and footless families of Brazil.

Three different studies have recently reported the correlation of birth deformities with ingestion of various tranquilizers by mothers in very early pregnancy. Meprobamate (the drug's name may be different on the bottle you're using — check with your doctor) and Librium (chlordiazepoxide) were implicated as causing various birth defects, but a fourth study of some 50,282 pregnancies failed to find any such clear association. A Finnish study also implicated meprobamate and further suggested that Valium (diazepam) taken in early pregnancy may be associated with a higher rate of cleft lips and/or palates. Corroboration comes from a study in Atlanta, Georgia, where Valium had been taken four times more often by women who had babies with cleft lips and/or palates than by those having babies with various other defects.

Another tranquilizer, Haloperidol, used in the treatment of schizophrenia and other agitated states, has been implicated as causing severe limb malformations.

For all these drugs and others, proving specific relationships to particular birth defects may be extremely difficult. Since there is rarely an urgent need to take these medications, they are best avoided when planning pregnancy or during the first four months.

Cortisone

Large numbers of pregnant women have taken cortisone. The general consensus at this time is that cortisone taken in pregnancy may be associated with a slight increase in birth defects. The problem is that the disorder for which it is given may be more important as a causal factor than the drug itself. Cleft palate is the most frequently reported defect.

Drugs for Diabetes Control

A variety of medications (insulin, tolbutamide, chlorpropamide, and others) are used for the control of diabetes. There is evidence to suggest that diabetic women have a somewhat greater (perhaps as much as two- or threefold) risk than nondiabetics of having children with birth defects. It is at present impossible to blame a particular drug used to control diabetes any more than the disease itself for birth defects.

Anticancer Drugs

In the late 1940s a certain drug called methotrexate was used in women with tuberculosis or cancer to induce abortion. It was discontinued after major defects of the aborted fetuses were noted. Subsequently, however, at least eight mothers are on record as having taken this drug to induce abortion. Some of these mothers failed to abort and gave birth to offspring with serious malformations, including severe bony defects of the skull (some bones missing), markedly malformed ears located low down in the neck, severe growth retardation, absent digits, and odd-looking faces. This drug continues to be used for both the treatment of leukemia and also for psoriasis. There are a number of other powerful drugs used to treat cancer, some of which have been associated with birth defects. Since it is uncertain whether any of these chemical agents cause a specific pattern of defects, that is, a recognizable syndrome, some of the disabilities may have occurred purely by chance. Nevertheless, there is an abiding need for women to be certain they are not pregnant when taking these and other powerful medications.

Drugs for Epilepsy

The question has repeatedly been raised concerning the possible adverse effects on fetal development of drugs, called anticonvulsants, used in the control of epilepsy. In this connection, a number of reports have described serious abnormalities such as heart defects, malformations of the brain and nervous system, intestinal malformations, mental retardation, defects of the genitals and urinary tract, cleft lip and palate, bone defects, and so on. Professor David W. Smith, in his studies in Seattle, has reported that about 11 percent of babies exposed to anticonvulsants (of the hydantoin group) while in the womb show minor and major birth defects and lower I.Q. scores than their peers.

Most recently, the reports indicate that the pregnant patient who is treated for seizure control runs a two to three times greater risk than a nonepileptic patient of bearing a defective child. Some reports point more specifically to particular drugs (e.g., Dilantin, trimethadione). Cleft lip with or without cleft palate seems to have been the most frequent abnormality observed in some studies, with a rate of 10 per 1000, compared to a rate of 1.5 per 1000 in infants of nonepileptic mothers. More work is still required, however, to establish clear cause and effect relationships between these drugs and the subsequent birth defects.

It is entirely possible that, at least in some of these instances, the epileptic disorder itself may be the causal factor through hereditary mechanisms. Moreover, during pregnancy the frequency and severity of actual seizures may damage the fetus by causing a lack of oxygen. It is also known that certain anticonvulsant drugs (e.g., phenytoin) may depress the body's immunity to infection. Theoretically, at least, women taking this medication subject themselves and their fetuses to a greater likelihood of infection. Certainly it is recognized that epileptics, probably because of the medications they take, have an increased risk of leukemia or lymphomas, both being cancers of the blood-forming cells. If you are a female epileptic, it would seem prudent to consider seriously with your doctor the need for any medication in early pregnancy. For seizure control, there may be no choice.

Sex Hormones

Sex hormones (progestogen and/or estrogen) may have serious effects on the fetus. One clearly established possibility is the masculinization of female infants, with the female genitals resembling those of a male. The male exposed in the womb may be born with an enlarged penis and scrotum, have pubic hair, be hyperkinetic, very aggressive, and resist sleeping during the first year of life. There is also some data that suggests that such males later on may be less "masculine": rated lower in aggressiveness and athletic ability when compared to their peers. Most recently, reports indicate a two- to threefold increase in the occurrence of heart defects following the use of sex hormones in early pregnancy. Other evidence implicates sex hormones with defective spinal vertebrae, anus, windpipe, esophagus, kidneys, and limbs. These last associations have yet to be established firmly. Women in early pregnancy usually take these sex hormone preparations in one of three situations. First, they may have been on an oral contraceptive that failed and become pregnant without realizing what had happened. Second, sometimes the sex hormones are used as a test to determine if a woman is in fact pregnant, thereby possibly setting up a situation where the fetus could be affected. Third, women who have had recurrent miscarriages take sex hormones to avoid having another one. In all three situations, the fetus may inadvertently be damaged.

Discussion of the diethylstilbestrol hormone disaster is taken up later in Chapter 19. Females who were exposed to the hormone while still in the womb fell prey to cancer many years later. Recently questions have arisen concerning the delayed effects of this hormone on males: one possibility being poor development and function of male sex organs.

Fertility drugs have come upon the scene in the last few years. They have been used to stimulate release of an egg or ovum from the ovaries. Women, trying for years to become pregnant, have received these drugs and found themselves pregnant with three, four, and even more fetuses. Some suspicion has developed that these drugs, Clomid (clomiphene) for one, may cause birth defects as well as multiple release of eggs. The difficulty in establishing any such association is that subfertility and abnormal fetal development may themselves be causally related in some way to birth defects.

Correlation between sex hormones and birth deficiencies is not easily proved, and at this time an absolute statement cannot be made, though the evidence is most suspicious, especially regarding heart defects. However, a large United States governmental study should report on its findings relatively soon. Meanwhile, prudence would dictate that women not take sex hormones in early pregnancy for any reason.

Anticoagulants or Drugs to Stop Blood from Clotting

Women in their childbearing years take anticoagulants most often for their varicose veins (deep vein thrombosis). There is evidence that these anticoagulants — and the drug Coumadin (warfarin) has been implicated — may cause birth defects that include malformation of the nose, abnormalities of cartilage, and mental retardation. Need I reiterate the plea that extremely careful consideration be given before taking any drug in pregnancy?

Drugs and the Thyroid Gland

Treatment of the overactive thyroid gland or hyperthyroidism during pregnancy is not a simple matter. The various drugs used may cross the placenta and affect the fetal thyroid, causing malfunction and possibly goiter. Excessive use of iodides in pregnancy, either as salts or because they're in cough mixtures and in drugs used for asthma, may also cause a large goiter in the fetus. There are cases where the thyroid was so big that vaginal delivery was impossible. Large goiters may compress the windpipe and kill the infant.

One source of iodide, often forgotten, exists in the compounds used for x-rays of the gallbladder and some other organs. Radioactive iodine, used to treat the mother's hyperthyroidism, may conceivably "wipe out" the fetal thyroid. The affected child might therefore be a cretin unless thyroid hormone is taken for life.

Smoking

A clearly demonstrated hazard of smoking in pregnancy seems to be the tendency to have smaller babies. We have detected the presence of nicotine and other substances resulting from smoking in amniotic fluid of smoking mothers as early as the fourteenth week of pregnancy. It might still be premature to conclude that smoking may cause no birth defects, especially when one considers that frequently multiple factors act together that could affect the fetus. While there has been some conflicting evidence about intellectual impairment in the children of smokers, who in addition suffer more often from respiratory disorders than the children of nonsmokers, it does seem clear that the smoking of over 20 cigarettes a day by a pregnant woman is associated with an increase in frequency of death in the first week of life.

LSD and Marijuana

Ingestion of LSD or other hallucinogenic drugs frequently causes fear of damage to the ovaries or testes and therefore to any offspring. As far as pure LSD is concerned, the evidence points away from any relationship to the birth of defective offspring. However, the presence of impurities in many of these hallucinogenic drugs poses unanswered questions. From a few reports in the medical literature, it is apparent that parents who have ingested these drugs have had babies with a number of birth defects. Because of the possibilities of impurities, no definitive and absolute answer can be given to prospective parents worried about genetic defects as far as future children are concerned.

I do not recommend amniocentesis and prenatal genetic studies in situations where ingestion of hallucinogens has occurred in pregnancy. If amniotic fluid studies in early pregnancy showed normal chromosomes, the fetus could still be abnormal. On the other hand, even if the chromosomes showed some breakage in the amniotic cells studied, the fetus could still be normal. In essence, then, if fetal abnormalities are caused by drugs like LSD, these defects are not presently diagnosable prenatally.

No solid evidence has been presented to indicate that marijuana smoking in pregnancy may lead to birth defects. Available studies do indicate that the active chemical principle in marijuana *may* have effects on the genes, may interfere with the response to infection, and possibly could have an effect on the fetus. The *potential* harm of marijuana smoking in pregnancy should be sufficient to dissuade a concerned couple from its use.

Poisons in Pregnancy

Alcohol is only jokingly called a poison, but could reasonably be so classified when considering its effects on the fetus. The likelihood of a baby of an alcoholic mother dying within one week of birth approaches 17 percent, which is remarkably high. Recently it was noted that women who are chronic alcoholics tend to have children with borderline to moderate mental retardation. A Seattle study showed that 44 percent of the babies of severe chronic alcoholics had I.Q. scores below 80, in contrast to only 9 percent with such scores in the matched children of nonalcoholics. A further 32 percent of the survivors of alcoholic mothers appear to have impaired growth, microcephaly, defects of the limbs, heart, joints, and usually minor abnormalities of the head and face.

In my view, the relationship of the abnormal features ascribed to maternal alcoholism still requires further study. It is
well known, for example, that a profoundly destructive atmosphere exists within the family with an alcohol problem, often
blighting the psychological and intellectual development of
the children. These psychosocial problems might well be the
cause of the developmental retardation (but not of the birth
defects), rather than the alcoholism itself. Nevertheless, I am
in agreement with the Seattle physicians in emphasizing that
parents, where the woman is the alcoholic, should consider
termination of the pregnancy because of the high risks of congenital defects and/or mental retardation. A woman who has
stopped drinking should probably take at least six months to
get her nutritional status and mental health back to normal
before conceiving.

Lead Poisoning

In 1971–1972, it was estimated that there were over 400,000
cases of childhood lead poisoning, leading to 150 to 200
deaths per year in the United States. While important steps
have been taken to combat these problems (mainly stemming
from lead-containing paint chipping off the walls and being
eaten by children), the problem has not as yet been irradi-
cated. Lead poisoning during pregnancy is decidedly rare
and fortunately so, because it has been known since the latter
part of the nineteenth century that stillbirth as well as congenital defects occurred in the offspring of mothers exposed
to high lead concentrations. More recently, however, it has
been noticed that the blood-lead concentrations in newborn
babies of mothers who live in high lead exposure areas (e.g.,
near expressways) may be elevated. Since it is known that
lead affects rapidly growing tissues, this observation is of some
concern. Furthermore, borderline increases in blood-lead
levels in mice have been associated with hyperactivity, and in
sheep with slow learning: two of our present educational
bugaboos.

Mercury Poisoning

You would not have thought that mothers are likely to ingest mercury during pregnancy, if at all. Tragic experiences, however, have occurred in both the United States and Japan, where pregnant women have ingested mercury contained in contaminated food and subsequently delivered severely malformed and retarded children. The Japanese episode occurred after a factory began discharging its waste into the sea adjacent to a fishing village. The high content of mercury in the factory's waste material soon contaminated the fish, which were caught by the local fishermen and eaten by them and their wives. Many families were affected, but it took about seven years before a connection was established between the ingestion by pregnant women of fish with a high content of organic mercury and the birth of children with severe brain damage and other defects. This disaster occurred in Minamata Bay and the condition was subsequently called Minamata disease.

The IUD and Copper

Contraceptive failure with the intrauterine device (IUD) may lead to pregnancy with the device in place. The copper from the IUD (which is the probable mechanism preventing implantation or survival of the fertilized egg) could conceivably damage the embryo. Indeed there has been an occasional report of serious malformations in the offspring of women who conceived with an IUD in place. No final statement can be made yet about the degree of risk in these pregnancies.

Occupation and Birth Defects

It is perhaps not surprising that certain occupations are associated with significant risks of having children with birth defects. You would most naturally think of those situations where the expectant mother is exposed. We have already described pregnant nurses who damaged their offspring by working in a nursery where a baby under their care was shedding rubella or other viruses. A similar risk situation applies equally to pregnant women physicians.

Certain male occupations have also come under suspicion. In at least two studies, men working with vinyl or polyvinyl chloride in fabrication industries lost many more offspring through fetal deaths than expected. Thus far the data have not shown a larger number of birth defects in *living* children of men working with these chemicals. The most likely mechanism for increase in fetal deaths is the vinyl chloride effect on the husband's sperm.

Very recently, observations have been made suggesting that medical and nursing staff working in operating rooms suffer an increased frequency of infertility, spontaneous miscarriages, and defective babies. Conclusions from a number of small studies in different countries have pointed in the same direction, although with different percentages of involvement.

The largest reported study was one done by the American Society of Anesthesiologists and reported in 1974. In that study, 49,585 operating room personnel were surveyed retrospectively and compared to 23,911 people who did not work in operating room surroundings. Females who were exposed to operating room conditions clearly experienced higher rates of spontaneous miscarriage, birth defects, cancer, and liver and kidney disease. Some of the increased risks were striking and most disturbing. For female nurse anesthesiologists, birth defects were up about 60 percent. Female physician anesthetists showed the same trend of increased birth defects in their offspring. Remarkably, even wives of male physician anesthesiologists had birth defects 25 percent more frequently than in the general population.

The best guess is that anesthetic gases are the causative agents. However, stress, which stimulates excessive hormone secretions, may possibly play some role here. Either way, there is sufficient evidence for a clear and distinct message. Women actually pregnant or perhaps even trying to become pregnant should absent themselves from the operating room throughout pregnancy. There is no solution, however, to the distressing dilemma involving the unexposed wives of exposed male operating room personnel, who also appear to have an increased rate of having defective babies.

Blighted Potatoes

A researcher in London in 1972 hypothesized that defects of the brain and nervous system, such as anencephaly and spina bifida, may be associated with the eating of blighted potatoes by pregnant women. His idea was that chemical substances from a specific mold infection of the potato could cause these defects in the developing embryo or fetus. His ideas met with a rather cool reception, but nevertheless led to potato-avoidance trials in a few centers. It soon became clear that even mothers who totally avoided potatoes throughout their entire pregnancy still had offspring with these defects. The current feeling is that the potato-blight hypothesis is not an acceptable explanation for the defects described above.

Drugs, poisons, toxic inhalants including tobacco, viruses, x-rays, noise, and a host of other agents constitute our environment. It is this environment that extends directly or via the placenta to the developing fetus. In particular, the dangers drugs spell are now perfectly understandable. In pregnancy, unless there are cogent medical reasons, only vitamins and iron in normal dosage are really safe.

CHAPTER 12

Genetic Counseling

GENETIC COUNSELING is probably as old as medicine itself. You will recall the accurate knowledge about hemophilia found in the Talmud. What is new about genetic counseling is the availability of options that never existed before. There is now the medical technology to prevent birth defects through prenatal diagnosis, to detect carriers of genetic disease though they have no obvious symptoms, to diagnose certain genetic disorders at birth, and to provide some specific treatments. These advances present you with vital options.

What It's All About

Genetic counseling is communication mostly between doctor and prospective parents and affected or concerned persons in reference to occurrence or recurrence of hereditary disorders. The aim is to provide those seeking information with the fullest understanding of the disease in question and its implications, as well as the options available. The counseling process aims to help families through their problems, their decision making, their possible anguish, and their adjustments. The goal is definitely *not* to make decisions for them.

The primary hope is that counseling will provide enough understanding to produce rational decisions that would serve to prevent or at least decrease the recurrence of serious genetic disease or mental retardation in a family. While a vast majority of counselors would agree with these goals and hopes in general, a variety of opinions exists about how genetic information should be obtained and conveyed, and even whether it should be withheld.

Who Needs Genetic Counseling?

The reasons why people seek genetic counseling can be grouped in general categories. They want to know 1. if they themselves have a genetic disease and whether they are carriers; 2. if they run the risk of having one (or another) child affected with a particular genetic disease; 3. what are the implications of a genetic disease already diagnosed as existing in one or both partners who are planning parenthood, and what is its prognosis and treatment; 4. what help can they get in making a decision about the options of prenatal diagnosis, selective abortion, artificial insemination by donor, or adoption; 5. what kind of help is available for their already affected child and where they can find it.

It would make sense for couples to seek counseling before or at the time of marriage, but certainly before conception — whichever comes first! In this way a child with birth defects would not have to be born to make them realize how they could have perhaps avoided it or at least benefited from prenatal counseling. Not infrequently, I have consulted with young couples contemplating marriage. A few of them have adopted a eugenic view: they broke off their relationships after hearing of their 25 to 50 percent risk of having seriously defective children with hereditary disease. That is mate selection on a true genetic basis: a practice that I suspect is still most unusual today.

In spite of all the new knowledge, at least 90 percent of the people in the United States, West Germany, and other Western countries who really need counseling do not receive it. This may be because they do not realize that a family disorder is hereditary, and their physician has failed to recognize it and neglected to refer them for proper advice. If you are worried about a particular family illness, that *alone* is sufficient reason to seek counseling. You will usually obtain answers and, more often than not, you will leave reassured.

Who Provides Genetic Counseling?

For the most common genetic disorders, experienced physicians may often be able to supply the needed information. For the rarer problems, consultation with a medical geneticist would be advisable, even if only for a second opinion. Very worried people may find their anxiety unrelieved after consultation with their own doctor. If he is sensitive to their unallayed fears, he should at least suggest a second opinion from a genetic specialist. Sadly enough, this seldom happens, and people remain anxious and possibly ill informed until crisis or trauma takes them in search of the necessary expert diagnosis.

Medical genetic counselors are usually pediatricians or internists who have concentrated on hereditary disorders. They often practice medicine or pediatrics in a major teaching hospital attached to a medical school. Most commonly, they operate as part of a larger team, some of them having more expertise in the laboratory than at the bedside. Many of the latter have earned graduate degrees. Members of such a medical team may also counsel. It would seem unwise, however, to be counseled, except perhaps on the most common, well-known genetic disorders, by someone whose experience has not been in the diagnosis, care, and management of disease.

Some genetic centers such as those at the Massachusetts General Hospital and the Yale–New Haven Hospital make it a practice to provide the patient with a written summary of the counseling provided. This is a useful technique, especially since some of the information may be both pertinent and critical to the children in the family. For example, if one or two of them are actual carriers of a particular genetic disease, then that information is critical to them when they marry and begin childbearing. This might be some 25 years later when the parents who originally went for counseling and the doctor have all died. The written summary is a valuable document and should therefore be kept with other important papers, such as the will or insurance policies.

The Counselor

Just as those seeking genetic counseling have a wide variety of backgrounds, personalities, beliefs, and so on, so do genetic counselors represent a wide variety of these features and therefore have many different approaches to the counseling process. The genetic counselor may be influenced by special eugenic views, religious beliefs, age, qualification, training, and personal prejudices, as well as the state of his or her physical and mental health.

Also, geneticists have differing perceptions of their obligations as counselors. The majority feel that their role is simply to provide as much information and understanding to the patient as is possible, making every effort to explore the disease in question in full, such as the prognosis, treatment and available options including artificial insemination by donor, adoption, prenatal diagnosis, and carrier detection. These counselors will also invariably discuss the implications of a genetic disease on the family and raise for consideration all issues of concern, including the religious views of the individuals, the economic implications or emotional burden of having an affected child, the possible effects on family life and on the other children, and the suffering or problems of an affected child. Moreover, they might be able to reassure the person who fears that there will be a social stigma attached to the disorder in question. Discussion of contraception and the effect of the whole problem on the parents' sex life may be raised, as well as the option of sterilization. Some counselors might even bring up the possible economic burden of the disabled child on society.

I recommend and practice the total communication approach. I believe that *everyone has a right to know and a freedom of choice.* All available information should be given out freely, the whole subject explored, and all matters of consequence discussed. The flow of information should not depend solely upon questions of those seeking advice. How could they, after all, anticipate the eventualities?

The Authoritarian Approach

A major difference of opinion exists among some genetic counselors with regard to method. The direct or coercive approach is to dictate exactly what to do or not to do, such as: do not have an abortion; have a vasectomy; arrange for artificial insemination; have a tubal ligation; adopt children; practice total contraception, and so on.

The danger of the directive approach is the insinuation by the counselor of his or her own religious, racial, eugenic, or other arbitrary beliefs into the counseling process. I have repeatedly seen physicians of certain religious persuasions counsel their patients to avoid prenatal testing and selective abortion. Some of these physicians of course argue that their advice is in the best interests of the family. Or, they may hold that the authoritarian approach is best because they maintain that so many parents are simply unable to comprehend all the factors and therefore cannot assess their risks and make the right decisions on their own.

Such an approach is, I think, to be condemned, not only on the grounds of counselor prejudice, but because it constitutes a moral affront to individual privacy. It is obviously a very personal matter whether you decide to have children or not, or to abort or not, and the doctor's role, in my opinion, is to provide you with all the information you could possibly need to make a balanced, rational decision on your own.

The noncoercive approach is not always easy, especially when the desire of a counselor to decrease the frequency of hereditary disease runs contrary to the desires of the parents. If the disease is a serious one, it is very tempting for the counselor to make every effort, albeit undictatorially, to persuade a couple not to have any more children. While this may be a valuable effort for the good of society at large and also might spare the family great unhappiness, it opens up opportunities for the counselor to insinuate his or her own religious, racial, or eugenic views into what should be objective counseling.

Not infrequently, patients ask the doctor to be "directive"

and to make a specific decision for them. "What would you do if *you* were in our position, Doctor?" I believe that every effort should be made by physicians not to succumb to the flattery of that question, but instead to spend more time with their patients, trying to help them discover their own priorities in life. It is neither practical nor right for a physician to extrapolate his beliefs, his life-style, and everything else onto his patients. His primary responsibility is to understand, diagnose, and give out all the information available from years of research and from his own experience.

What Should You Look for in a Genetic Counselor?

What you expect may be very different from what others are searching for. A major factor is the degree of your personal involvement. If you were inquiring about your risks of actually having Huntington's chorea, though it had not yet made itself evident, your anxieties would be very different from those of someone, prior to finding a mate, simply trying to determine if he or she were a carrier of some genetic disorder. Should you have a child with muscular dystrophy or cystic fibrosis, then your desire for advice and treatment might assume proportions of desperation. Or, in contrast, you are adjusted to the idea of a hereditary disease in your family and, having just married, are calmly considering your options.

The decision to seek genetic counseling may be one of the most important decisions of your life. This means that extreme care should be taken in choosing a genetic counselor. You are looking, ideally, for *knowledge* and *humanity*. You want not only expertise, but someone who is sensitive, aware of your anxieties and fears, and willing to give you an empathetic hearing. The best counselors know how to face a wide range of expectations, of educational levels, and different religiously and emotionally oriented personalities.

The best counselor also communicates in a nontechnical language that is easily understood. The problems are often complex, and patience here is not only a virtue, but an absolute requisite. Consultations must take time; they cannot be rushed. You have a *right* to expect such treatment.

Expectations of the Counselor

While you may have defined expectations, so do counselors. A very important one is that both members of a couple, when appropriate, come for counseling together. The complex issues of guilt, culpability, family prejudices, serious differences of opinion between the spouses, pervasive ignorance and fear — to mention only a few — make this very important, if not mandatory. No letter can replace face-to-face discussion. Moreover, with the emotional chaos so often present, the problem of incorrect interpretation of the information to the absent spouse and the possible lack of appreciation of the true risk situation should make it abundantly clear that a couple come for counseling together. Then your expectations and those of your counselor are more likely to be fulfilled.

Risks and Odds

As he proceeds, the counselor must take cognizance of a whole host of factors. Simply telling the parents that they have a risk of recurrence for anencephaly of 3 to 5 percent in every subsequent pregnancy does not mean the parents have understood or grasped the degree of probability. Some parents might regard a 5 percent risk as almost no risk at all, while others might consider it so grave that they decide to have no further children. Explanations that a hereditary recessive disease has a recurrence risk of 25 percent might be totally misinterpreted. It means that for *every* pregnancy there is a 25 percent risk of the particular disease occurring again, and this risk does not change with the number of children already born, affected, or unaffected. Some parents may make the mistake of thinking that since their first child already has the disease, they will be safe in their next three pregnancies! We have all, unfortunately, seen the consequences of such misunderstanding by parents.

Chance, Indeed, Has No Memory!

To complicate matters even further, it is recognized that the appreciation of risk and the interpretation of odds vary among basic personality types. A pessimistic parent may reach conclusions very different from those of an optimistic parent with the same odds in mind. A basic difference in the attitude toward risk between achievement-orientated and failure-threatened persons is also well known. Moreover, attitudes toward risk do change with changing moods.

The Anxiety Block

Genetic counseling in the presence of overwhelming anxiety never proves to be very useful, since most of us have difficulty in assimilating all the information communicated by a doctor in moments of stress. Recognition of this anxiety block by both doctor and patient is very important and is best handled by scheduling a return visit some weeks later to re-explore all the issues, questions, and answers discussed in the first session.

Besides anxiety, denial of a diagnosis by one or both parents may serve as an even greater roadblock. Mothers may refute the fatal prognosis or possibly insist that the disease in question is not even hereditary. I have even seen one father, unable to accept the information that he was a proven carrier of a genetic disease, deny that he was the father of the child!

Other Obstacles

Recently in an important study at Johns Hopkins Medical School, imperfect reception of genetic counseling was noticed in some 44 percent of the families under observation. That same study confirmed what all of us have known or suspected for years: religion is the principal obstacle to the intelligent use of genetic research. For various religious reasons, many couples, regardless of the high risk of producing a child with a serious or fatal genetic disease, simply push ahead having more and more children.

The counselor is also faced sometimes with difficult intra-family problems that complicate the counseling process. You will recognize that, in your own family or in others, communication between members is often disappointingly minimal or absent entirely. You may know families, as I do, where the parents elected not to tell their children about their first deceased child, or that there is still an older brother or sister with severe mental retardation tucked away in some institution. I recall one twenty-year-old patient complaining bitterly that when she was on the point of marriage she discovered through a neighbor that she had a brother, defective from birth, still living in an institution. Her parents had hidden this information from her for the twenty years of her life. Suppression of the truth is not only morally questionable but may even have legal implications. We have seen women who chose not to inform their sisters that they too ran the risk of having a child with a serious sex-linked disease such as muscular dystrophy or hemophilia.

Where to Go for Genetic Counseling

I have already suggested that the ideal genetic counseling is obtained from a team of experts located in a major hospital/medical school complex. This ideal situation, like so many others in life, is not easily found. Nevertheless, there are many excellent centers providing genetic counseling, in many instances supported by the National Foundation–March of Dimes. And don't forget that your own pediatrician or internist may be able to provide you with all the information you need.

CHAPTER 13

Artificial Insemination by Donor: An Option

ONE OF THE IMPORTANT OPTIONS offered in genetic counseling is artificial insemination by donor or AID. It is not a new idea or technique, mentioned as far back as in the Talmud and in steady use since the end of the eighteenth century at least. An estimate in 1957 suggests that up to that time, worldwide, there had been about 100,000 births due to AID. More recent estimates credit it with some five to ten thousand births per year in the United States.

Who Needs AID?

Infertility in the Male

Couples who have tried for a few years and failed to establish a pregnancy may be candidates for AID, though it would of course first have to be shown that the male and not the female partner has the problem for it to be a sensible option. Approximately 12 percent of all married couples are infertile (some estimates suggest that this amounts to about 2 million couples in the United States), with the male partner being responsible about 10 to 15 percent of the time. We will not discuss the gynecological reasons for infertility, nor the medical problems involved in male infertility or sterility. Suffice it to say that if the semen contains an insufficient number of sperm or the quality of the sperm is low (for example, the sperm swim poorly), AID can be considered.

Ejaculation of semen in man may under some conditions occur in a retrograde fashion: that is, the semen being released into the bladder and not out through the penis. While this so-called retrograde ejaculation occurs only infrequently, it may be one of the rare causes of infertility, especially in diabetes mellitus. It is known that ejaculation is controlled usually through the brain but may on occasion be a completely reflexive action (for example, ejaculation may often accompany judicial hanging). Techniques are available to manage cases of infertility caused by retrograde ejaculation. In 1971, Dr. Richard B. Bourne and his colleagues first described the successful and most unusual use of artificial insemination in a case of retrograde ejaculation.

The patient was a thirty-three-year-old man who had been diabetic since the age of eight years, and blind for three years. He had married four years previously, and he and his wife complained of their inability to establish a pregnancy. So far as he could remember, he had been unable to ejaculate since the age of twenty-five years, although his orgasm had been normal.

Retrograde ejaculation was confirmed by noting the absence of semen in a condom after intercourse and then seeing sperm in the first urine specimen passed after coitus.

On the day his wife was due to ovulate, a catheter was inserted through his penis into the bladder in order to wash it with a special sugar solution. The catheter was removed and the patient then allowed to ejaculate, the semen being obtained by having him urinate as soon as it was possible after ejaculation. The urine sample containing the semen from the bladder was then spun in a centrifuge, and the semen (which collected at the bottom of the tube) was drawn into a syringe and used to inseminate his wife.

This procedure was repeated about eight times over a six-month period without success. Finally it was realized that the urine was too acid — sperm do poorly in an acid medium. His urine was thereupon alkalized by a dose of sodium bicarbonate on the evening before and the morning of insemination. This technique succeeded, and his wife duly became pregnant and delivered a normal baby girl.

One unusual indication for AID arose during the Vietnam War when some Californian wives were inseminated by sperm from their husbands overseas.

AID for Genetic Disorders

When the male has a serious disease like Huntington's chorea, and he and his wife therefore run a 50 percent risk in every pregnancy of having an affected child, AID can be a godsend. Even if the male has not yet shown any signs of the disease, but knows that he *may* later in life, artificial insemination is sometimes chosen in order to safeguard the offspring.

A male with hemophilia would pass the gene to all his daughters, who would then be carriers and transmit the disease to half their sons, another example of a need for artificial insemination.

AID is also important as an option when both parents are carriers of some autosomal recessive disease such as cystic fibrosis or sickle cell anemia. It should be realized, however, that simply by chance, the donor of the sperm might coincidentally be a carrier of the disease in question. (As we have said, about 1 in every 25 whites is a carrier of cystic fibrosis.) If prenatal diagnosis is possible for one of these recessive disorders, and a couple are not against abortion of a defective fetus, then AID is not necessary.

Blood Group Incompatibility

Parents with incompatible blood types, especially those involved in the Rh negative problem, are specific candidates for artificial insemination by a donor. We have noted, from time to time, women spontaneously aborting severely affected fetuses pregnancy after pregnancy, then suddenly having a perfectly normal baby. It took no geneticist to guess that the woman had solved her problem and achieved insemination that was not artificial.

The Sperm Donors

Selection

Most frequently, sperm donors are medical students or young physicians in training, all of whom are known to be of normal intellectual capacity and in excellent health. Usually a careful family history of the donor is taken in order to diminish the chance that he could transmit a genetic disease, though testing to determine if he is a carrier of any specific disorder is not done. The physical features of the donor, including aspects of his complexion, hair, eye color, stature, and so on, are noted in order to match him to the recipient parents. His blood type is determined and his semen is examined a few times to check the count and quality of the sperm. Usually donors who are continually available to provide semen, even on weekends, are selected. Most commonly, they are paid $30 to $50 for each semen sample provided. Some view the payment of sperm donors as unethical, while others feel that such inducement may lead to the concealment of pertinent family history about genetic disease. They point out that blood from paid versus voluntary blood donors is of lesser quality and is infected more often. Tests to ensure that donors do not have venereal disease are not invariably performed,' but should be. The anonymity of the donors is assured by a code system, which further enables use of the same donor for insemination of other patients. There is obviously a theoretical chance that children born into different families through artificial insemination from the same donor may marry each other many years later. This would really amount to marriage between a half-brother and a half-sister. The risk in such unions for having offspring with serious genetic disease (see discussion on incest, Chapter 6) would be very significant, but if you're concerned about the offspring of AID marrying, contemplate for a moment results of some studies made in England and the United States that show about 30 percent of children in certain areas are conceived through adultery! The risks that these children might ultimately marry half-brothers or half-sisters would seem to be distinctly greater than the risks of AID offspring intermarrying.

The Infertile Couple

Many couples who might benefit from AID simply do not approach their physician because of the inability of one or the other to handle the emotional aspects. Usually the woman is extremely motivated to have a baby and is willing to go along with it. Many men, however, are unwilling to go this route. There appear to be many reasons, the most common of which relate to the male's confusion between infertility and sexual inferiority. He may feel that his virility is at stake. The matter of personal pride, aesthetic distaste, or moral aversion may be other reasons for not wishing AID.

All couples who approach a physician for AID are carefully interviewed together, and the insemination procedures and methods of donor selection are explained. Special care is taken to indicate to the male that having insufficient numbers of sperm or sperm of inadequate quality to effect fertilization has nothing to do with his sexual prowess or performance. If the couple are perfectly cognizant of all the issues involved, as well as the possible marital, psychological, and legal implications, then both are asked to sign a document to initiate the proceedings. This document absolves the sperm donor of responsibility for paternity, and also absolves the physician of any responsibility for subsequent birth defects or problems during pregnancy and delivery. The couple are, of course, assured of complete privacy and confidentiality. The sperm donors as well as their wives waive all rights to the resulting children. Moreover, they also waive the right to any legal action to discover the identity of the infertile couple. Some physicians even mix sperm from a few donors, so that the true biological father can never be known.

Occasionally, it is necessary for the couple to receive counseling from their clergyman, a psychologist, or a psychiatrist if they are ambivalent about the whole process. Generally speaking, most physicians are unwilling to provide AID to infertile couples unless both partners are explicitly keen on it and no marital instability is evident. In this context, it is striking that even after the thousands of babies conceived in this way, the child's paternity has rarely been an issue in marital breakups.

Success with AID

The fullest cooperation from both parents is required to ensure the maximum chance of establishing a pregnancy. Very careful psychological evaluation of both prospective parents is necessary prior to initiating AID. Generally the overall success rate ranges between 60 and 85 percent, though it may take six to eight months to achieve a pregnancy. Nevertheless, persistent failures do occur in at least 15 to 20 percent of patients. As for birth defects in the offspring conceived through AID, available data suggest that the frequency is somewhat lower than average. If this is true, it might reflect the careful selection of at least one set of parental genes. It should also be emphasized that the other viable alternative to AID is adoption, and this should always be fully explored with every couple.

Sperm: Fresh or Frozen?

The use of either fresh or frozen semen for AID is possible. Obviously, having to have a group of individuals constantly "on call" to provide semen samples is not the best method, especially when trying to inseminate a woman who ovulates erratically. Techniques have thus been evolved to freeze away semen samples in liquid nitrogen at temperatures of minus 196°C. In this way, samples are readily available and can be used repeatedly in the same patient daily or more often if necessary. There has been no clear evidence thus far to indicate whether fresh or frozen sperm is the more successful method.

A useful aspect of frozen semen storage is that it can be

utilized in men whose sperm counts are low but not zero. Semen samples from an infertile male could be pooled in order to raise the total sperm count and then utilized for insemination of his wife. There are other situations that have arisen where the frozen storage system is useful. Men undergoing vasectomy may wish to store a number of semen samples as a form of "family insurance," which would ensure that they could still father offspring in case of marital breakdown or death of their children. Rarely, prior to x-ray therapy for treatable types of cancer where it is possible that the testicles may be exposed, the male decides to provide a series of semen samples for storage, in case he should be rendered sterile after the irradiation therapy.

AID and the Law

Clearly all the participants in artificial insemination are subject to legal purview: the donor, the recipient female and her lawful husband, the physician involved, and finally the child born as a result.

It was only as recently as 1968 that the California state supreme court decided in a unanimous opinion that a child conceived through AID with the knowledge and consent of the woman's husband is truly the legitimate offspring of that marriage. Other states have followed suit. No American court, to my knowledge, has found AID to be an adulterous process. In fact, a court in Scotland, as far back as 1958, concluded that AID even without the husband's consent was not adultery and not even grounds for a divorce.

The recognition that a child born following AID is legitimate has been crucial since illegitimate children may not be able to inherit and have no right to claim the necessities of life from their nonbiological fathers. This is an important point in the instance of divorce, where one or more children have been conceived by AID. Claims for financial support from the mother's ex-husband, who is actually not the father of the child, have been repeatedly upheld in court.

Physicians providing AID should secure evidence that the couple are truly married, that the marriage is not subject to annulment, and that the couple are living together. The couple must provide written consent to the procedure and a signed agreement to raise any resulting children as their own.

Should the child conceived through AID be told how he was conceived? You're aghast even at the possibility! Well, ponder the question as you consider this case. A certain boy's father was dying slowly from a dementing hereditary brain disease (Huntington's chorea). The boy became extremely distraught because of the 50 percent chance that he had for developing the same disease. To avoid a nervous breakdown, the boy's mother told him that he had been conceived through AID because his father, aware that he had the disease, had chosen to protect his future children by arranging for artificial insemination. Not only was the boy incredibly relieved, but he also expressed deep warmth and gratitude toward his dying father.

A number of other perplexing questions in this field remain either unclearly answered or not answered at all. Now with the increasing recognition of women's rights, may an unmarried woman be inseminated? May a married woman seek and obtain AID *without* consent of her husband? Finally, is the use of frozen sperm subject to regulations governing human experimentation? While AID remains an important option for infertile couples or those selecting the technique because of genetic disease problems, a certain degree of religious, moral, or social conflict is bound to remain.

CHAPTER 14

Prenatal Diagnosis:
Amniocentesis

"DOCTOR, IS MY BABY NORMAL?" The universal question of hope and uncertainty. A plea for a happy beginning. Virtually every woman worries during pregnancy, hoping and praying that the baby she will have will be normal and healthy. This anxiety is shared to a greater or lesser extent by the father of the expected child. We are all comforted by the knowledge that about 96 in every 100 babies are born *without* major birth defects. But the 3 to 4 percent of babies who are *not* born sound are the root cause of our anxieties during pregnancies.

Indeed, many informed couples today sensibly concern themselves about their risks of having a defective or deformed child *before* they start a family, having become aware that it is possible, in an increasing number of situations, to prevent tragedies.

This chapter introduces you to what is at present your main option in the prevention of birth defects, mental retardation, or genetic disease. This option is *prenatal diagnosis:* a technique that allows for the accurate diagnosis of serious or fatal genetic disease in the fetus early in pregnancy. Once such a diagnosis is made in the fetus, you may choose to have an abortion and try again with another pregnancy. Dozens of questions must be running through your mind. How are these prenatal tests done? When? Who needs to have such studies? Who does these tests? Where? Are they accurate? You're opposed to abortion — what if the fetus is defective? I will try to answer most of the questions you are likely to be thinking about in a sequence of four chapters on prenatal diagnosis, concluding with a discussion of some of the overriding moral, ethical, legal, and social issues in Chapter 17.

Background Developments

The diagnosis of genetic disease in the fetus has only a very short history. During the early thirties it became possible to introduce a needle into the womb to sample the fluid in which the fetus grows. Some three decades later, in 1961, the first diagnosis of a genetic condition was made with the fetus still in the womb. The disorder was that of Rh incompatibility between fetus and mother, which could possibly result in the death of the fetus or newborn baby from hemolytic anemia. Research made rapid advances in the understanding of this disorder, which was first treated in the early sixties by exchanging the blood of the fetus still in the mother's womb with blood of the correct blood group. Subsequently it became possible to prevent this disorder by immunizing susceptible mothers who were Rh negative. Studies on the fetus with blood incompatibility problems are, however, confined to the *last 3 months* of pregnancy. In contrast, prenatal studies to detect (and increasingly to treat) other serious genetic diseases are done between *14 to 16 weeks of pregnancy.*

The ability to determine the sex of the fetus by simply staining a cell was first successfully applied in 1955 to cells from the amniotic fluid derived from the fetus. This work had been based upon the serendipitous though critical observation made by Dr. Barr and Dr. Bertram in Canada, in 1949. They had been studying the nerve cells of cats and noticed that after staining with certain dyes, cells from the female had a darkly stained blob on the outer edge of the nucleus. This blob, subsequently called the Barr body or chromatin mass, was not present in male cells, thereby allowing us for the first time to differentiate male from female cells by means of a very simple technique. In 1960, success was achieved in demonstrating the fetal sex in pregnant women who ran the risk of having children with sex-linked disorders (affecting males only) such as hemophilia or muscular dystrophy.

In the mid-1960s, technological developments in actually growing human cells in laboratories made it possible to analyze the chromosomes in cells from the amniotic fluid as well.

Experience in diagnosing diseases using chromosomal analysis slowly began at that time. In 1968, Dr. Carlo Valenti, in New York, first diagnosed a fetus with Down's syndrome (mongolism). Since then, testing the fetus for genetic disease has gradually become widely available. Let us examine the current situation in detail.

Counseling Before Amniocentesis

Ideally, each woman having an amniocentesis for prenatal genetic studies should be counseled before the procedure. This may simply be done in a careful discussion with her obstetrician, *with* her husband present. Such arrangements are probably acceptable if the amniocentesis is for a routine hazard such as advanced age of the mother. The obstetrician should of course be expected to know the risks of the procedure and be able to discuss all the relevant aspects.

When the disorder in question is rare or complicated (such as the biochemical disease galactosemia), a consultation with a medical geneticist is advisable. An obstetrician is not expected to know the various types of this disease, how it is treated, what the chances are for mental retardation, and how abortion could possibly be avoided. Many disorders *cannot* be diagnosed through amniocentesis, while in others, tests for carriers may make the procedure unnecessary. Consultation with a medical geneticist in these types of disorders, as well as others, obviously makes a lot of sense.

Informed Consent

Amniocentesis is of course a minor surgical procedure, and as such requires prior consent. In agreeing to undergo the procedure (as would be the case for elective abortion), the physician is required to inform the patient carefully about the very small risks of the test. In addition, both he and the laboratory doing the studies should ensure that the couple involved know that the removed cells may not grow in the laboratory in 5 to 10 percent of cases, that a second or even third amniocentesis may be needed, that the answers provided are not 100 percent guaranteed, and that *other* genetic disorders or birth defects will *not* be excluded by the test. Moreover, the result provided from one fluid pertains only to one of the pair should twins be present. In my unit, written consent is also required.

What Is Amniotic Fluid?

A few days after fertilization of the egg by the sperm, the new embryo attaches itself to the wall of the womb. The embryo becomes enveloped in a thin-walled sac. This sac — very much like the yolk of an egg — slowly fills with fluid secreted mainly by the embryonic and, subsequently, fetal tissues. Ultimately, fetal urine adds to the volume of fluid within the sac inside the womb. This liquid is the amniotic fluid in which the fetus is suspended and grows.

At the site where the embryo attaches to the womb, a circular, flat structure develops, called the afterbirth or placenta, which serves as a direct communication between the fetus and the mother. The placenta, while being a safety barrier to some of the toxic agents eaten by the mother, also does let through nutrients, infectious agents, and certain drugs such as aspirin, for example. At the same time, some substances from the mother's circulation also contribute to the amniotic fluid of the fetus. The amniotic fluid contains a variety of chemical substances including proteins, carbohydrates, and fats as well as cells that originate from the fetus.

How Are the Studies Done?

The amniotic fluid contains cells that peel off the skin of the fetus or are passed from inside the mouth or lining of the lung through the intestinal tract or in the fetal urine. When these cells are examined after the amniotic fluid is obtained for study, some are found to be dead. Many, however, are living cells, and it is these that we are able to grow in our laboratories. These cells are placed in sterile dishes or flasks containing a rich broth and kept in a warm incubator in the laboratory. The broth is changed a few times a week, and the growth of these cells is observed closely under the microscope. One cell divides into two, then from two into four, from four into eight, and so on, until there are thousands to millions. This usually takes two to three weeks, at which time the cells are broken open in order that their chromosomes can be examined. A cell has to be in a particular phase of division, called metaphase, when the chromosomes are spread out, for the examination and chromosome determination to be successful. Between 15 to 30 cell "spreads" are usually examined in each case. With these techniques, then, it is possible to determine the chromosomes of the fetus, the sex, and the activities of a whole array of different enzymes.

A result is generally obtained from the first amniotic fluid in about 90 to 95 percent of cases. Nevertheless, a number of things may go wrong along the way. The obstetrician obtaining the fluid may be careless and use an unsterile bottle for the amniotic fluid or contaminate the sample as it is squirted into the container. The laboratory personnel may also contaminate the sample when feeding the cells. In my laboratories, total loss of a sample because of contamination is extremely unusual (only 4 times in the first 1000 cases!).

Even without contamination the amniotic fluid cells may simply not grow. This happens in 5 to 10 percent of cases. A repeat amniocentesis because of a failed cell culture then becomes necessary.

Some physicians do not ensure safe delivery of the sample to the laboratory, but I feel the patient should be certain that due care will be taken for its transport. Generally the best results are achieved when the sample reaches the laboratory within hours of its being obtained. It should then be worked on, and if possible not left overnight. Where there is no choice, the sample may be left in a refrigerator (4°C) overnight. We have, on occasion, successfully grown amniotic cells sent to us from countries 10,000 miles away, having been five days in transit. Bloody amniotic fluid samples are obtained in about 10 percent of cases, but this will not usually hinder the study, except perhaps to slow down cell growth a little, unless the sample is extremely bloody.

How Amniotic Fluid Is Obtained:
Amniocentesis

The procedure to obtain amniotic fluid from the womb with a small needle is called amniocentesis (see Figure). It is usually performed by an obstetrician, who first administers a local anesthetic into the skin somewhere between the pubic hairline and the navel, before inserting the needle into the womb (some women prefer to have the needle inserted only once, and do not even have the local anesthetic). The amniocentesis is performed in the doctor's office or on an outpatient basis at the hospital. The recommended time for the procedure is when the mother is between 14 to 16 weeks pregnant. The reason for this timing is that the enlarging womb emerges from the pelvis into the abdomen of the pregnant mother at 12 weeks of pregnancy. Before that time, it cannot be felt through the abdominal wall. Between 14 to 16 weeks, the womb can easily be felt between the pubis and the navel. Therefore, it is relatively easy to insert a needle into the womb at this stage of pregnancy.

The Use of Sound Waves

We routinely recommend that ultrasound or sound wave test studies precede the amniocentesis. This technique, which is safe, involves the passage of high frequency sound waves through the womb and makes it possible to locate the placenta accurately. In this way, the needle can be inserted into the womb, avoiding the placenta, thereby decreasing the chance of bleeding. Unfortunately, in 40 to 50 percent of cases, the placenta lies along the front wall of the womb, and the needle must pass through it. The ultrasound study also enables one to measure the diameter of the fetal head and possibly diagnose a gross brain defect (anencephaly), a very large head (hydrocephalus), or a very small head (microcephaly). Repeated ultrasound studies, every few weeks, may be valuable in trac-

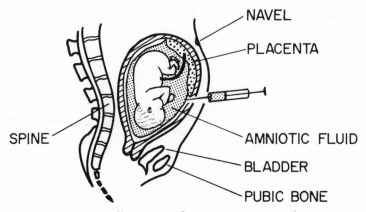

NAVEL

PLACENTA

SPINE

AMNIOTIC FLUID

BLADDER

PUBIC BONE

Amniocentesis needle entering the amniotic cavity without pene-
trating the placenta.

ing the expected normal pattern of head growth. Such measurements also allow for continual assessment of fetal body
growth, since some hereditary disorders are often correlated
with poor fetal growth, called intrauterine growth retardation.

Most importantly, perhaps, ultrasound can be used to detect
the presence of twins or triplets (see Chapter 16). If the amniocentesis is done without prior ultrasound and therefore without knowing that twins are present (twinning occurs in about
1 in 80 pregnancies), serious consequences may ensue. The
parents may be running a high risk (25 percent) of having a
defective child, and if the twins lie in 2 different sacs, only one
amniotic fluid is obtained with the needle. The result then
pertains to only one twin *unless* ultrasound studies are used.
Usually twins are diagnosed much later in pregnancy. One
mother, who had had a previous child with severe mental
retardation due to a biochemical genetic disease, discovered
ten weeks after her amniocentesis with a normal result that she
was carrying twins. At 29 weeks of pregnancy, too late for
more testing or for abortion, she became agitated and depressed
because there was no information about the other twin, who
could have been affected. This mother was fortunate in that
both children were normal and healthy at birth.

I am aware that ultrasound machines may not be available in small towns or rural areas. Even in the big cities many amniocenteses are done without prior ultrasound. This clearly is not the ideal, but some doctors argue that the needle has to pass through the placenta anyway in 40 to 50 percent of cases. I feel that when the risk of having a defective child is high (say 10 percent and over) ultrasound studies are mandatory, and the patient should travel to a major center for that purpose.

Time and Timing

At present, to determine the chromosomes of the fetus, two to three weeks on the average are required before the results become available. For some of the rarer hereditary biochemical diseases, up to six weeks may even be necessary. It is therefore important that the amniocentesis be done at the best time, which is from 14 to 16 weeks of pregnancy, to provide early reassurance or an opportunity for the parents to elect abortion. Many sad experiences have occurred when this test has not been done at the right time. In one case, the amniocentesis was done at 28 weeks of pregnancy, and a seriously defective fetus was diagnosed at 30 weeks — much too late for abortion. While carrying this fetus for another 10 weeks, the mother developed serious depression and threatened suicide. She duly delivered the defective fetus as predicted.

While there have been some instances where the physician forgot to offer the amniocentesis either at all or too late, much more often the pregnant woman comes for her *first* obstetric visit *too late* in pregnancy. In many cities, for example, women may seek their first appointment with the doctor when they are almost five months along. If families are concerned about having children with birth defects, they should arrange their first pregnancy visits no later than *directly* after the *second* missed period.

How Safe Is Amniocentesis?

Obstetricians have been performing amniocenteses for decades. Almost 45 years ago, substances were being injected into the amniotic fluid for fetal x-ray studies. The most common reason today for a pregnant woman to have an amniocentesis is for the management of blood incompatibility (Rh disease). Tens of thousands of amniocenteses have been performed on women in the last three months of pregnancy in the course of managing Rh disease, with complications to the mother or fetus occurring only rarely.

It would be reasonable to believe that inserting a needle into the womb does carry some hazards for both mother and fetus. Theoretically, at least, it may be possible to pierce a blood vessel and cause some bleeding, to introduce infection, or to precipitate premature labor and therefore cause a miscarriage, or to damage the fetus. Certainly, no accurate figure has been available until recently about the risk of amniocentesis for genetic studies.

In October 1975, the United States federally funded National Institute of Child Health and Human Development Collaborative Amniocentesis Registry Project reported its findings after a four-year study. Nine collaborating centers, including my own, had studied 1040 women who had amniocenteses and another matched group of 992 women who had not undergone amniocentesis. Care was taken to match women for many important differences, such as age, the number of previous pregnancies, race, income group, husbands' occupation, level of education, and so on.

Those women who had amniocenteses had no major complications themselves. Some women had minor "complications" that included transient cramps, vaginal spotting (bleeding), or leakage of a little amniotic fluid.

There was no significant difference in miscarriage or fetal death in women who had had an amniocentesis compared to those who had not. Analysis of the data confirmed an observation made in Chicago by Professor Henry Nadler, of North-western University School of Medicine, before the four-year collaborative study began. This was that women having amniocenteses had a *lower* rate of miscarriage than those who did not have the prenatal diagnosis procedure. But one must take into account the likelihood that women having amniocenteses are better informed, take better care of themselves, choose their doctors more carefully, and their doctors in turn are probably more up-to-date and practicing better medicine.

Even though the Collaborative Amniocentesis Registry Project observed no increased risk to a pregnancy because of amniocentesis, my experience (involving even more cases) suggests that there is a slight risk of miscarriage, albeit very small: less than 0.5 percent or 1 in 300 to 400 at most.

No significant damage to the fetus was observed in babies whose mothers had amniocenteses, although a skin scratch or puncture mark by the needle was possibly noticed in one case. The Collaborative Amniocentesis Registry Project analyzed the babies born in both their control groups again at one year of age, and no differences in the frequency of birth defects or motor/mental retardation were found. The conclusions of this careful collaborative study indicate that amniocentesis is a safe though not completely risk-free procedure. Similar studies in Canada and England have come to the same conclusion. By the way, it also became clear that about 3.2 percent of women who do not go through the testing nevertheless miscarry or have a fetal death during the last six months of pregnancy.

A Balance of Risks

How would you decide whether the slight risk in amniocentesis of causing fetal loss or damage was outweighed by the risk of having a defective child? This decision making could be described as balancing chances, or more properly, a balancing of benefits. If, for example, the mother is aged forty and pregnant, the approximately 3.4 percent chance of fetal chromosomal disorder is between seven to ten times the chance of miscarriage through amniocentesis. In this situation, parents are likely to opt for the latter. If the mother is between thirty-five and thirty-nine, the risk of having chromosomally abnormal children (e.g., mongolism) approximates 2.2 percent. She therefore is about four to six times more likely to have a chromosomally defective child than to miscarry as a result of prenatal testing. However, the decision of a couple who have been trying for a pregnancy for five to ten years may obviously differ from that of a couple who already have had six children. The worry about losing the long-awaited offspring would likely dominate the decision of the first couple.

Who, then, most needs amniocentesis and prenatal studies? The Rh negative sensitized mother with an Rh positive husband is naturally going to need help. There is, however, a large group of mothers whose plight is more subtle and less well known. We will devote the next chapter to them.

CHAPTER 15

Prenatal Diagnosis: Chromosome Disorders

THERE ARE MANY reasons why you (or your spouse) should consider prenatal genetic studies. You may have a family history of a certain hereditary disease, a previously affected child, or had repeated miscarriages, you may be over thirty-five, and so on. The reasons for prenatal studies can be grouped in four general categories: couples at risk for having a child with 1) a chromosomal abnormality; 2) a sex-linked disease; 3) one of the hereditary biochemical disorders of metabolism; 4) a hereditary disfiguring birth defect. In this chapter we will only consider the chromosomal disorders category.

Certainly the most common reason anywhere in the world for prenatal studies is to determine the chromosomal constitution of the fetus. And small wonder, since in every 200 children born in Western countries, 1 has some chromosomal abnormality — close to 20,000 in the United States alone. On the other hand, it is remarkable to what extent nature takes care of its own mistakes through the process of miscarriage (see Chapter 2).

Between 40 to 60 percent of all fetuses studied after miscarriage show serious chromosomal abnormalities. Those miscarried in the fourth month have been found to have them in 25 percent of the cases; after four months in only 3.5 percent of cases. Careful analyses of infants dying within days of birth reveal that about 5.6 percent of them have chromosomal disorders. Our bodies, it would seem, have a mechanism to counteract such errors, though they slip up from time to time. But now with the help of advanced medical technology, what nature has overlooked can be diagnosed early in pregnancy.

It is true that the only sensible option for prevention of the effects of chromosomal error is termination of the pregnancy.

But you or your spouse may be against abortion and even prenatal tests, and you have a right to reject them. Equally, if you have no such aversions and the fetus is known to be defective, you also have your rights: to terminate the pregnancy.

I reiterate: the decision to abort is *solely* a parental one, which should remain as uninfluenced as is humanly possible by the physician or anyone else.

Frequency of Chromosomal Disorders When the Mother Is over Thirty-five

For reasons that are not yet exactly understood, older mothers give birth to children with chromosomal abnormalities much more often than younger mothers. Women pregnant when they are between thirty-five and thirty-nine years old run a risk of about 2.2 percent of producing a child with abnormal chromosomes. The risk continues to rise: from about 3.4 percent at forty to around 10 percent when the mother is over forty-five years old. The number of previous children born to these mothers does not affect the risk figures.

Both patients and doctors alike have associated this risk mainly with Down's syndrome or mongolism. But though this is the most common disorder, *four other* chromosomal disorders are also correlated with increased maternal age.

Nowadays, in the United States, between 5 to 6 percent of all pregnant women are thirty-five years of age and over, giving birth to more than 160,000 babies each year. Of all babies born with Down's syndrome, about 25 percent are delivered by women who are thirty-five years and over.

Although I have been recommending amniocentesis for pregnant women of thirty-five years and over for about seven years, the vast majority of them have ignored this option. In 1974, I reported that in Massachusetts only 4.1 percent of them had studies done. The percentage was estimated to be even lower in most states of the Union.

There are probably many reasons for this remarkable underutilization of a relatively new but very important technique.

When the aforementioned United States government-funded Collaborative Amniocentesis Registry Project (see Chapter 14) made its report in October 1975, many physicians were still concerned about the safety and accuracy of amniocentesis. Some were not familiar then (and perhaps even today) with the indications for prenatal studies. Others were against abortion. Also, facilities for testing during the late sixties and early seventies were not available in many states.

Today, with the safety and high accuracy of prenatal diagnostic studies well documented, there would seem to be little reason why all women who need them should not get them. But, alas, the facilities are now found wanting, in that there are insufficient trained personnel (laboratory technicians) or laboratories in the United States and elsewhere to provide these crucial services. What is required is the appropriation of sufficient funds to establish adequate services. In the context of federal health money disbursed, the sums required are relatively small. This matter requires urgent government attention. Major United States population centers are simply unable to provide the testing service to many couples who need it. The grave impact of all this becomes more meaningful if you were the person denied these studies because of the lack of facilities, and unnecessarily had to give birth to a profoundly retarded child. Every couple in or entering their childbearing years and other concerned people should press their legislators for immediate action on funding such services.

Parents Who Are Carriers of Chromosomal Abnormalities

Most of us really don't know if we are carriers of a chromosomal abnormality. Certainly at least 1 in 1000 people do carry such abnormalities, which when transmitted to their offspring could result in birth defects and mental retardation (see Chapter 2). Since population testing for chromosomes is currently not feasible, the only reason you might consider having a blood test is because of a family history of chromosomal abnormality, including a previously affected child.

If a child has Down's syndrome due to an extra # 21 chromosome, then blood tests of the parents are usually not obtained. If the child has a chromosomal translocation or mosaicism (see Chapter 2) then the parents' blood is tested to determine from which side of the family the problem may have originated. Once that is established, brothers, sisters, and other relatives on that side of the family can be tested. Prenatal genetic studies are best offered in subsequent pregnancies where one parent has been shown to have translocation. In about 2 percent of infants with Down's syndrome, one of the parents is found through chromosomal studies to be a carrier of the translocation abnormality. Since these hereditary forms of chromosomal abnormalities can be diagnosed in the fetus, most of these parents can, through prenatal diagnosis, avoid the birth of an affected child.

The importance of acting on the knowledge about the family history is exemplified by one recent case of mine:

Joanne was eighteen and unmarried. When she found herself pregnant by her fiancé she came for genetic counseling. Her pregnancy had already advanced to 16 weeks. The reason for seeking counseling was that her sister had Down's syndrome. She was therefore worried that her child might inherit it. It was not known at that time which kind of Down's syndrome her sister had: the very uncommon hereditary form or the common nonhereditary type.

Because there is a very significant risk of carrying a fetus with Down's syndrome for those individuals who carry the hereditary form of mongolism, amniocentesis and prenatal genetic studies were provided immediately.

Some two weeks later, when the results came in, it turned out that her fetus had the hereditary type. This eighteen-year-old prospective mother and her fiancé then elected to have an abortion, which was done forthwith and the affected fetus found as predicted. Blood studies for chromosomal analysis on her, performed prior to abortion, had shown also that Joanne was a translocation carrier of the disease, and later we

confirmed that her sister and mother were carriers of hereditary Down's syndrome too.

Less than one year later, now married, Joanne again presented herself for prenatal studies — this time three months
pregnant. At the recommended time (14 to 16 weeks of pregnancy) an amniocentesis was performed. We were able to
show on this occasion that the second fetus had normal chromosomes and was a male.

On the very day that this normal result was provided, she
indicated that she had been exposed to what sounded like
classic German measles when she was three months pregnant.
Immediate blood studies disclosed that she had indeed contracted the infection. Therefore, another amniocentesis was
performed between 21 and 22 weeks of pregnancy and the German measles virus was found in the amniotic fluid cells. The
parents elected — for the second time — to abort this pregnancy as well. Studies on the aborted fetus showed severe
fetal infection by German measles virus, confirming the prenatal diagnosis. As we have said, children born after rubella
infection in the womb may have major birth defects including
mental retardation, cataracts, heart defects, stunted growth,
and deafness (see Chapter 10). (Amniocentesis is not usually
recommended for mothers who are not immune to rubella and
have been exposed to it while pregnant.)

Some months later she arrived with a third pregnancy. Amniocentesis this time revealed one amniotic fluid cell with a
ring-shaped chromosome (which is decidedly abnormal) in
about 60 cells analyzed. We indicated that we (and others)
did not know the meaning of this observation and did not
believe it likely that the fetus was affected, but could not be
sure. The young couple, having already been through so
much, decided to keep the pregnancy. They had their daughter as predicted, and she looked like a sound baby. Chromosome studies on both blood and skin revealed a normal
pattern!

A Previous Child with Down's Syndrome (Mongolism)

Parents who have had a child with the nonhereditary form of Down's syndrome (trisomy 21) have a 1 to 2 percent risk of having another similarly affected child. But I have personally seen at least a half dozen families who originally had a child with nonhereditary Down's syndrome and subsequently had another similarly affected baby. Amniocentesis is therefore always recommended if the parents have had a child with trisomy 21.

Miscellaneous Reasons for Prenatal Chromosome Studies

Many problems brought up most often by young couples are not considered suitable for prenatal studies. If either the mother or father have experimented with hallucinatory drugs, or if the mother has been a heroin addict and is now being treated with methadone, amniocentesis is not recommended. Nor are prenatal studies suitable at this point for patients exposed to rubella, chicken pox, other infectious diseases, or even radiation during pregnancy. As explained in Chapter 10, our present inability to provide a reliable diagnosis makes the testing neither feasible nor sensible.

Women, however, with overactive thyroids are justified in seeking prenatal studies because of the evidence suggesting that they may have an eightfold risk of bearing offspring with some sort of chromosomal abnormality. Women with underactive thyroids similarly have an increased risk.

Also, in the case of a woman bearing twins, there is, according to studies done at Yale, a sixfold risk that one member of the pair will have a chromosomal abnormality. Occasionally it may be known that one of the parents of an expected baby has unusual and abnormal chromosomes. This will increase the hazard to the child, and amniocentesis and prenatal studies are clearly indicated. If the mother has suffered recurrent miscarriages, there is a small, though definite, chance (3 to 8 percent) that she or the father will be found to have a minor but significant chromosomal abnormality (see Chapter 2).

The young pregnant mother who requests an amniocentesis on the basis of anxiety (her neighbor may have just given birth to a child with mongolism) does not usually get one: the policy at most centers is to provide prenatal studies only to those who run a well-determined risk. Indeed, some of the centers do not have enough facilities to deal with the women in urgent need. We are obviously years away from the ideal situation. It is, sadly, mainly a question of economics.

Accuracy and Errors

Data from the United States Collaborative Amniocentesis Registry Project found an accuracy rate for prenatal studies of 99.4 percent. This was based on some 6 cases out of 1020 in which an erroneous diagnosis was made.

In three of these, the fetal sex was determined incorrectly, mainly because diagnoses were offered before a sufficient number of cells were available for study. It was not a serious matter, in that none of the three couples ran any risk of a sex-linked disease.

Sad to report, however, there were two cases in which normal chromosomes were reported, but later infants with Down's syndrome were born. In one of these, it is entirely possible that the sample of amniotic fluid sent to the laboratory belonged to another patient who was having an abortion on the same day.

The inaccurate diagnosis in the sixth case was of a biochemical disease, galactosemia, for which treatment is available. The parents luckily elected against abortion. Soon after birth, the baby was found not to have the disease!

In my estimation, the error rate in the United States is about 7 per 1000 cases, most being mistakes in determining the sex of the coming baby. Considering the accuracy of laboratory tests in general, prenatal genetic studies achieve a high score.

Errors have been and probably will continue to be made. Parents must bear this in mind when deciding whether to have amniocentesis or not. An important factor is the choice of a laboratory that has sufficient experience in prenatal diagnosis.

CHAPTER 16

Prenatal Diagnosis:
Hereditary Disorders of Males,
Other Biochemical Diseases,
and Disfiguring Birth Defects

THE CHROMOSOMAL DISORDERS we just discussed are generally associated with risks appreciably below 10 percent. In contrast, the risks of having children with the disorders we are about to discuss are much higher and range between 25 to 50 percent. If you were faced with a 25 to 50 percent risk of having a child with a serious or fatal genetic disorder, you might, as very many prospective parents have done in the past, have chosen not to have any (or any more) children.

Since 1968, prenatal diagnosis of these more complex disorders has become of critical importance. It allows parents the opportunity of selectively having unaffected children, sparing them the agony of losing a child, and, more importantly, sparing the affected child the pain and suffering of early death, disease or deformity.

Our discussion is best divided into three categories of disorders where prenatal diagnosis is important:

1. Sex-linked disorders
2. Hereditary biochemical disorders
3. Hereditary physical birth defects

Prenatal Studies for Sex-Linked Disorders

We discussed sex-linked inheritance in Chapter 2 and noted that sex-linked diseases occur in males only, while in some *sex-limited* diseases, females only may be affected. There are about 150 recognized sex-linked diseases affecting each organ system. For example, there are sex-linked diseases of the brain, blood, skin, eyes, and so on. Among these many sex-linked diseases, only four are found in which the prenatal diagnosis can specifically be made. They are individually rare and are named after physicians who described them: Fabry's disease, Hunter's syndrome, the Lesch-Nyhan syndrome and Menkes' steely-hair syndrome.

Fabry's disease is really a biochemical disorder caused by a missing enzyme. A complex fatty substance accumulates in the body because of the missing enzyme (which would ordinarily break this compound into pieces) and causes kidney and blood vessel problems leading to high blood pressure, kidney failure, and strokes. Most patients in the past, after many years of symptoms, have died in their thirties and forties due to a lack of specific treatment. The question is, if you were the parent, would you elect to terminate a pregnancy in which the fetus was diagnosed as having Fabry's disease?

Hunter's syndrome is also a biochemical disease with a missing enzyme, and this time the complex substance that accumulates is called mucopolysaccharide. Accumulation of this material in all parts of the body leads to multisystem problems. For example, deposits of this substance in the brain will lead to mental retardation, in the heart to cardiac failure, in the joints to severe limitation in movement, in the liver to marked enlargement, and so on. Death in almost all patients occurs invariably by the twentieth year, and usually much earlier, after prolonged suffering. Unlike Fabry's disease, one cannot lead any sort of a normal existence in the intervening years before death.

The Lesch-Nyhan syndrome — also a biochemical disorder with a missing enzyme — is an extremely unpleasant disorder characterized not only by profound mental retardation and features of brain damage (stiff limbs with peculiar movements), but also by self-mutilation. Indeed, some of the patients whom I have seen have so severely bitten themselves around the mouth and limbs that I and other physicians have been left in a state of shock upon realizing that these were self-inflicted injuries. These patients may live on many years in their profoundly retarded state, given good care and attention. They often require restraining (for example, tying up their hands) to prevent them from mutilating themselves.

The fourth sex-linked disorder specifically diagnosable in a male fetus is one called Menkes' steely-hair syndrome. Affected children with this disease have hair that feels similar to steel wool and, in addition, they are retarded. The basic defect in this condition concerns the way the body handles copper!

Except for these four mentioned sex-linked disorders, none of the other diseases in this category can now be diagnosed in the fetus. This limitation, I'm happy to say, is slowly beginning to change. At present, the only recourse the parents have concerning sex-linked diseases is to determine the sex of the fetus. If a female fetus is found, the parents can be reassured. However, if it is determined that there is a male fetus present, then there is a 50 percent chance that that male fetus is affected. Since there is no way of being certain, the parents must decide simply on the basis of the high risk whether to take a chance or terminate that pregnancy. Consider for a moment the unusual plight of Sharon:

Sharon was twenty-six, unmarried, and four months pregnant when she came for genetic counseling. She had had one son from a previous pregnancy, who had been affected by a disease of his immune system (inability to fight infection). He died in infancy from overwhelming infection. Thereafter, she had been counseled that this disease was sex-linked, which meant that she was the carrier, and that every time she had a male child, he would have a 50 percent chance of having the disease. She simply refused to accept that she was "responsible" and consequently sought out a different father for each of her next two babies.

For the second pregnancy, she again refused prenatal studies and had a baby boy who also died from infection during the first year of life.

Her third partner convinced her to have prenatal studies in her third pregnancy. This she eventually did, and the results *showed a female fetus. This time she gave birth to a healthy girl and married the father.*

There are some unusual sex-limited diseases that are confined to females. Disorders of this kind (e.g., incontinentia pigmenti — a skin disorder associated with brain damage) are managed by determining whether the fetus is a female. In this group, virtually all females will be affected, and the parents could selectively elect to have normal boys.

Hemophilia and muscular dystrophy are two of the more common sex-linked diseases that are familiar to most people. But there are so many others that great care must be taken by both the doctor and the family in obtaining an accurate family history. Renpenning's syndrome, in which there is mental retardation without any other physical signs, is confined to males. I well recall one family — whom I saw before the days of prenatal diagnosis — in which the child being examined already had two brothers with mental retardation and three mentally retarded uncles with the same disorder. The only way to suspect sex-linked inheritance is for the physician to carefully analyze the family pedigree. Increasingly it is possible to perform tests to detect the carrier of such diseases. It is now possible in over 90 percent of cases to detect the carrier of hemophilia by a blood test. This represents a new advance. About 75 percent of carriers of muscular dystrophy can also be detected by a particular blood test. Unfortunately, the carrier detection tests for both hemophilia and muscular dystrophy do not provide answers in 100 percent of cases, and a negative result causes uncertainty and leaves the question basically unanswered. Fortunately, carrier detection tests are steadily becoming possible in more of the sex-linked and other disorders.

Prenatal Studies for Hereditary Biochemical Disorders

Many hundreds of different hereditary biochemical disorders of metabolism are known. Some estimates suggest that 1 in every 100 children born has one of these biochemical disorders. Many of them do not cause mental retardation, or impair the child's normal development or general health to any extent, or even at all. However, many cause severe mental retardation, seizures, stunting of growth, and early death. Close to 80 of these biochemical disorders can now be diagnosed in the affected fetus early in pregnancy (see Appendix II). The first biochemical disorder to be diagnosed in the fetus while in the womb was only made in the late sixties and was Tay-Sachs disease.

How Are the Diagnoses Made?

Cells from the amniotic fluid are placed in small dishes containing a nutrient broth, and kept in a special warm moist incubator. They grow slowly, and after a period of 3 to 4 weeks (occasionally as long as 6 weeks) there are enough cells to work on. Each of the cells having the genetic blueprint will show up the specific biochemical defect (e.g., deficient activity of an enzyme), thereby enabling a diagnosis to be made. The major problem in this group of disorders is being able to grow sufficient cells. Not infrequently a second amniocentesis may be required.

It's obviously wonderful news to hear that the fetus does not have the particular biochemical disease in question. But could you imagine the dismay if the child, instead, had Down's syndrome. I therefore feel strongly that once the suspected biochemical disease has been excluded, the chromosomes also be studied from the same sample.

Who then needs an amniocentesis and prenatal genetic biochemical studies? There are presently three clear indications:

1. Where both parents are found to be carriers of a particular hereditary biochemical disease in which accurate prenatal diagnosis is possible. The best-known example would be Tay-Sachs disease, where prospective parents may have been tested in a communitywide screening program. A number of couples where both were found to be carriers

have been identified before they had any affected children. They subsequently had each pregnancy monitored by prenatal studies, invariably opting to terminate pregnancies when an affected fetus was diagnosed. In this way, these couples were spared the torture of having a child develop normally for six to eight months and then begin to retrogress and deteriorate, having seizures, going blind, being in a vegetative state, wasting away, and dying usually between two and five years of age.

Knowledge that someone may be a carrier may only be discovered when his/her sibling has an affected child, and he/she goes to have tests done.

2. When the parents have previously had a child affected by a biochemical genetic disorder that can now be diagnosed prenatally.

3. Where carrier detection is either inconclusive or impossible in parents at risk, but where the prenatal diagnosis can be accurately made.

Treatment in the Womb

The primary goal of making an early prenatal diagnosis is to treat the fetus successfully while in the womb. Aborting the whole organism is obviously not the ideal approach, though it is the only way available at present for the vast majority of serious/fatal genetic diseases.

For a few disorders, treatment of the fetus directly (Rh disease) or through the mother has now succeeded.

At the Tufts University School of Medicine, Professor Mary Ampola, aided by colleagues at Yale, made the first prenatal diagnosis of a *biochemical* disorder called methylmalonic aciduria, *treatable* in the womb. This disorder in the fetus causes failure to thrive, vomiting, lethargy, biochemical disturbances, poor muscle tone, and eventually mental and motor retardation.

They treated the fetus through the mother during pregnancy by giving her intramuscular injections of massive doses of vitamin B_{12}. In this way, the child was well at birth and has continued to be well, taking a special diet (low protein) throughout her first three years. There have been no serious problems, and mental retardation and possible early death were averted.

Galactosemia is another treatable, hereditary biochemical disease where prenatal diagnosis is possible. If the fetus is affected, special dietary (lactose-free) treatment of the mother started early enough will almost invariably avert early death or mental retardation, cataracts, and liver damage. There are a few other disorders (such as some vitamin-dependent diseases, the adrenogenital syndrome, and hypothyroidism) where prenatal diagnosis may be critical to save life or prevent mental retardation or other consequences. Progress in actual prenatal treatment for genetic disorders can be anticipated, provided that fetal research is not even further interdicted by state legislation. A few other disorders are now being conquered by early diagnosis and treatment in the womb. Continued support for medical research will undoubtedly provide more and more opportunities for early treatment or prevention, reducing the need for abortion — the major option today.

Prenatal Studies for Gross Physical Birth Defects

The defects in this category — and there are very many — are gross physical deformities for the child. In these cases, the chromosomes appear normal, and no biochemical deficiency can be demonstrated. Typical abnormalities in this group are those with missing or deformed hands or limbs, gross malformation of the head (anencephaly), very big head (hydrocephalus), heart defects, and scores of other anomalies. Five approaches are useful in tackling the prenatal diagnosis in this group of diseases.

Sound Waves (Ultrasound or Sonar)

The use of sonar has moved from a research and development phase to accepted use as a new diagnostic tool (see Chapter

14). This technique involves the passage of sound waves through the uterus, thereby enabling accurate measurement of the fetal head size and hence its age, location of the placenta, detection of twins or triplets, and diagnosis of some major disfiguring defects.

If twins are detected by sonar, and the risks of genetic disease are high (i.e., over 10 percent), it is possible to outline one amniotic sac by instilling a radio-opaque substance into the amniotic fluid through the amniocentesis needle. Under x-ray and sonar control, amniotic fluid can be obtained from the second sac. Technologically this is a difficult procedure, the reliability and safety of which are yet to be shown. In the presence of multiple fetuses, a high genetic risk, and an inability to obtain fluid from both sacs, the parents may have to decide on keeping or terminating the pregnancy based on the statistical risks of genetic disease alone.

If twins are detected before the amniocentesis, parents should give extremely careful consideration to the next step: the actual amniocentesis. Amniotic fluid from one sac will be obtained, studied, and a result provided. What if the fluid around the other twin cannot successfully be obtained? The first result may be normal, but what then if the other twin is abnormal? Or vice versa? It is extremely rare (but not unheard of) for both twins to be affected, but not unusual for one to be affected. The dilemma is not eased, because the option to terminate the pregnancy may mean abortion of a normal fetus! (See Chapter 14, p. 158.)

The prenatal diagnosis of malformation of the brain and head or anencephaly has been made in early pregnancy by the use of ultrasound. The same technique has also successfully been used in the prenatal diagnosis of polycystic disease of the kidney in later pregnancy. Neither hydrocephalus nor microcephaly — both very often associated with mental retardation — have yet been diagnosed in the fetus early in pregnancy. Theoretically, the prenatal diagnosis of both these disorders may be possible at least in some cases by serial measurements at two- to four-week intervals till twenty-four weeks of pregnancy.

Special X-ray Techniques

This procedure — called amniography or fetography — involves the instillation of a contrast solution through a needle directly into the amniotic fluid. The contrast medium adheres to the skin of the fetus, thereby allowing a very clear silhouette to be seen on x-ray. Thus, a grossly abnormal head, an abnormal spine, gross limb deformities, or absent limbs can be visualized. Some success has been reported with the use of this technique in late pregnancy, but there is still little experience between 16 and 24 weeks of pregnancy — the time when prenatal diagnosis may really be most helpful. Because of the small experience with this technique in the fourth, fifth, and sixth months of pregnancy, no idea of the degree of risk involved has yet emerged (see also Chapter 10).

X-rays

The bone structure of the fetus is at a very early stage of development around 16 weeks of pregnancy. Therefore, there is a very limited use of x-rays to visualize bone abnormalities. Between 20 to 24 weeks of pregnancy it is possible to obtain, in some cases, useful diagnostic information. For example, there is one serious hereditary bone disease called osteopetrosis in which the bone density is greatly increased. The prenatal diagnosis of this disease has, in fact, been made at least once at 24 weeks of pregnancy using x-rays. Theoretically, at least, other serious hereditary bone diseases in the fetus may be diagnosable in the same way. I would recommend special heed be taken of your family history before seeking this kind of study.

Biochemical Studies on the Amniotic Fluid

As mentioned in Chapter 14, the amniotic fluid contains a large variety of different chemical substances that, in the main, are derived from the fetus. One of these substances is a particular kind of protein made by the fetal liver and called alpha-fetoprotein. In 1972, it was first noted by researchers in Scotland that the concentration of this protein in the amniotic fluid was very much elevated when the fetus had a severe malformation of the brain (anencephaly) or of the spinal cord (spina bifida or myelomeningocele).

This protein is made by the fetal liver, secreted into the fetal blood stream, excreted into the fetal urine, and then into the amniotic fluid when the fetus urinates. When there are "open" defects of the brain, as in anencephaly, or of the spine, such as spina bifida or myelomeningocele, the alpha-fetoprotein leaks out directly into the amniotic fluid, thereby raising the concentration of this protein. By simply measuring the concentration of alpha-fetoprotein in the amniotic fluid, it is possible to diagnose prenatally about 90 percent of these defects. None of these was diagnosable in pregnancy prior to 1972. About 10 percent of these defects (most frequent in people of Irish descent, see Chapter 6) are covered by skin and do not allow the leakage of alpha-fetoprotein through into the amniotic fluid; this test is not useful in these cases. Ultrasound and amniography can often be utilized to diagnose this group. But despite the utilization of all techniques currently available, there will still be a few remaining fetuses, amounting to a small percentage, where the defect is so small or flat that no current prenatal technique is able to discover it. Some of these very small undiagnosable defects are, however, remediable by surgery soon after birth.

Experience has, unfortunately, shown that this new biochemical test, while representing such a major advance in making the prenatal diagnosis of grave nervous system disorders, is really nonspecific. That is to say, there are some other conditions in which a raised alpha-fetoprotein level is found. Perhaps the most common situation is where the fetus has actually died or is in imminent danger of dying. Most of the other conditions with raised alpha-fetoprotein in the amniotic fluid occur only rarely (such as congenital nephrosis).

Because the concentration of alpha-fetoprotein is high in the fetal serum, any fetal blood obtained inadvertently during amniocentesis may cause a rise in the level of alpha-fetoprotein found in the aspirated amniotic fluid. Ultrasound studies are therefore especially critical since they may help prevent bloody "taps" by enabling the obstetrician to avoid needling the placenta. False-positive results, a high alpha-fetoprotein level being found when the fetus does *not* have a defect, may create a problem. In fact there have been a few cases where perfectly normal fetuses have been aborted because of the concern and anxiety of the parents about the meaning of the elevated alpha-fetoprotein level. In my laboratories, the chance of a false-positive alpha-fetoprotein result is now about 1 in 1000.

It has also been discovered that when there is a high alpha-fetoprotein level in the amniotic fluid, this protein leaks into the mother's blood circulation. Theoretically, it would therefore be possible to take a blood sample from the mother between 14 and 20 weeks of pregnancy and, by looking for alpha-fetoprotein, discover if her fetus has an open defect of the brain and nervous system. These studies have been initiated in England, in our laboratories, and elsewhere. Preliminary data are showing that it is indeed possible to detect between 90 to 95 percent of pregnancies where the fetus has anencephaly, and close to 90 percent of cases when the fetus has spina bifida, by simply taking a blood sample from the mother and measuring it for alpha-fetoprotein concentration. An elevated level would lead to the recommendation of a more accurate diagnostic amniocentesis. Much work must still be done before this test can become part of routine antenatal care. These studies have important personal and public health implications because between 6000 to 8000 affected children are born each year in the United States alone. These defects occur in 1 out of every 500 births and therefore are among the most common birth defects seen.

Fetoscopy

This technique involves looking directly at the fetus through a tiny telescopelike instrument whose caliber is the size of a large hypodermic needle. This fetoscope, as it is called, is introduced into the uterus via the abdominal wall under local anesthesia. This procedure is still in the research stage of development, but represents an important advance in prenatal diagnosis. The first technique used was to insert a needle into the placenta and obtain fetal blood. This was first achieved experimentally in pregnancies just prior to elective abortion. Most recently, by obtaining fetal blood directly, the prenatal diagnosis of a serious hereditary hemolytic anemia, thalassemia, has been made. This disorder occurs most commonly in people of Mediterranean descent (see Chapter 6). In the same way, the prenatal diagnosis of sickle cell anemia has been achieved.

Clearly much more research will be necessary to develop the instrumentation and technological expertise as well as the safety of this procedure. Success with this effort, however, would clearly revolutionize all efforts at prenatal diagnosis. Having fetal blood for chromosomal analysis would, for example, provide an answer in three to four days instead of close to three weeks or more. Some biochemical disorders could be diagnosed on the same day the fetal blood is obtained instead of waiting almost six weeks. The benefits to anxious parents of early treatment when possible, or quicker action if pregnancies require termination, are obvious.

The second significant contribution of fetoscopy will be the ability to examine the outward appearance of the fetus. In this way, it may well be possible to diagnose prenatally gross physical abnormalities such as cleft lip and palate, missing or abnormal ears, deformed or absent limbs, spine abnormalities, and so on.

Exploring "inner space" has been an exciting and demanding challenge. Using very small caliber fetoscopes, only small areas of the fetus have been observed in one visual field. For example, we could see the ear perfectly well, but because of the rigid nature of the instrument being used, have had difficulty in negotiating around the head to visualize the face. The other frustrating problem is that the fetus suspended in fluid moves, and it is difficult to follow with a rigid instrument. Of course, the more instrumentation used and the longer the time spent maneuvering inside the uterus, the more likely is the pregnancy to be disrupted by miscarriage. Work is currently in progress in a few centers around the world to develop more sophisticated instruments. Legislation in some states (e.g., Massachusetts) has seriously impeded progress in fetoscopy.

Diagnosing Fetal Disease Through the Mother

There are a few disorders of the fetus that can be diagnosed by actually testing the mother — without an amniocentesis! Rh incompatibility is the best known. In another disorder, methylmalonic aciduria (see p. 176) examination of the mother's urine may alert the doctor to the disease in the fetus.

Most recently, the knowledge that fetal blood cells cross the placenta into the mother's blood stream is being utilized. A team at Stanford University in California led by Professor Leonard Herzenberg has pioneered a device called a cell sorter. Among the cell sorter's possible functions is the ability to sort through millions of the mother's blood cells for the relatively few fetal blood cells in her circulation. Should they prove successful, it could mean prenatal diagnosis for many disorders without an amniocentesis. There are, unfortunately, still considerable technical hurdles to overcome before this exciting tool can be applied in any routine way.

The prenatal diagnosis of hereditary disorders has represented the most significant advance ever in the prevention of mental retardation and serious/fatal genetic disease. There are many hereditary disorders, however, that cannot yet be diagnosed prenatally, and it is important for all prospective parents to recognize such limitations. Meanwhile, and for the foreseeable future, many parents facing genetic risks are and will be blessed by healthy children whom they would otherwise not have had at all. These opportunities and options are due solely to the advances in prenatal diagnosis.

CHAPTER 17

Ethics, Morality, the Law, and Prenatal Diagnosis

THE SIGNIFICANT CLINICAL BENEFITS of every major advance in medical research have inevitably raised social and legal issues. Kidney and heart transplantations are but two recent examples. The "new genetics," best exemplified by prenatal diagnosis and carrier detection, has, as expected, made waves disturbing both the family and society at large. The acceptance of these new genetic advances depends enormously on personal belief and morals and equally on theology and the laws of the land. Questions and dilemmas have arisen. The impact has fallen on parents, physicians, the fetus, and on our social institutions.

The Parents

All parents, given the choice, would undoubtedly choose to have a child who is normal and healthy. No such choice, however, existed until the late sixties when it became possible to predict accurately whether or not the fetus had certain serious genetic defects early enough for the parents to elect abortion if a fatal or untreatable defect was found. When the United States Supreme Court decision in 1973 made abortion legal, the last obstacle was removed in making the crucial prenatal diagnosis test a practical option for parents.

A Prior Commitment

There are parents solidly opposed to abortion, who would rather not know whether the fetus is defective or not. Others, concerned about the morality of abortion, often have an amniocentesis and prenatal studies anyway, hoping that no defect will be found and that the question of abortion will not come up. Some centers have declared that no amniocentesis would be provided unless the parents made a *prior* commitment to abortion if the fetus were found to be defective. This I believe to be entirely unwarranted, since all parents have a basic *right to know,* not only about their own personal health, but also about the health status of their future child. Centers insisting on this prior commitment point to the time, effort, hazards, and expense involved in prenatal genetic studies, stating that these limitations do not justify them in providing answers that will be ignored. In my laboratories, my philosophy has been to allow studies on all those at risk wishing an amniocentesis *without a prior commitment to abort.* Those parents who are ambivalent do not invariably have to address themselves to the question of abortion. When confronted with the bad news that the fetus indeed has a serious genetic defect, most parents nationwide have opted to terminate the pregnancy.

Abort a Defective Fetus?

The *fundamental* philosophy of prenatal diagnosis is to *reassure parents at risk* that they may *selectively* have *unaffected children.* In only about 3 percent of all at-risk pregnancies studied is a fetus found so defective that mental retardation or serious/fatal genetic disease is certain. Hence, only about 3 percent of all cases studied end up with considering and usually choosing an abortion. However, *because* of prenatal diagnosis, thousands of couples, who were too petrified to take a chance on account of their risks, now have their own healthy children. Indeed, *more couples are now able to have children because of prenatal diagnosis and only occasionally have to terminate a pregnancy.*

Those who would rather take high risks of having a defective child than abort have every right to stick to their beliefs, though they may agonize through the rest of their lives with the knowledge that they have condemned a child to pain, deformity, and possibly the horrors of institutionalization. (I cannot help but reiterate here the opinion handed down by the Rhode Island Supreme Court that "a child has a legal right to begin life with a sound mind and body."

One might expect that those individuals who choose not to abort obviously defective fetuses would themselves take care of their suffering offspring, who leak feces and urine, can *never* be toilet-trained, are blind, deaf, profoundly retarded, and have to be attended day and night. You might be amazed to find how many families who are "morally" against abortion place their children in institutional situations equal to a horrible living death. This also, I guess, is their right.

I have so often seen the misery, despair, and absolute desperation of parents trying to take care of extremely defective children in their homes. Yet those who institutionalize their children are almost invariably wracked by guilt. Either way, I believe in respecting their right to choose. I definitely do not subscribe to the view held by an increasing number of people that parents who elect not to have prenatal diagnosis, and subsequently have children with defects that could have been prevented, should be financially responsible for the care of such children. (Their point is that sooner or later we all pay through taxes for the care of the defective.) I do believe, though, that prospective parents should pause to reflect on the future that stretches ahead of them before turning down prenatal diagnostic studies. But, as I have said, I do not believe it is the responsibility or the right of either the physician or society to "tell" the parents what to do.

Wife vs. Husband

Difficult situations have arisen where a father, against abortion, has found himself in disagreement with his wife, who wishes to abort a defective fetus. You can imagine — if you have not already seen it — a woman who is a carrier of a sex-linked disease, such as muscular dystrophy, deciding that she will not continue the pregnancy if the fetus is a male, while her husband, believing he is the decision maker, insists that the pregnancy not be terminated. The courts have already addressed this question and, in Illinois, recently denied a husband's motion to prevent his wife from having a routine abortion. The court declared the right of privacy "was broad enough to encompass a woman's decision whether or not to terminate her pregnancy." This stand is in accord with the established legal principle that every adult of sound mind has a right to determine what shall be done with his or her own body.

Determining the Sex of the Fetus

Many laboratories, including our own, have been approached repeatedly for prenatal sex determination on the basis that if the fetus is not of a particular sex, then abortion would be sought by the parents. I have taken the position that prenatal sex determination for "family-planning" reasons really represents an inappropriate use of a very scarce and expensive technology, and have therefore always declined to provide any such service. This action that I have taken is indeed counter to my fundamental philosophy that parents have a right to know everything about their fetus, including its sex. However, when faced with the fact that in the United States alone, close to 200,000 women require prenatal studies annually for advanced age or other handicaps, and that in 1974, only about 3000 were studied, I have no hesitation in limiting the services to those who are at risk.

The Physician

A Matter of Trust and Communication

On occasion, the parents of an affected child may expressly forbid their physician to contact or communicate with other family members, who may be at risk for possibly having offspring with the same disease. In muscular dystrophy, for instance, the mother's sisters may have an increased risk of being carriers.

Would you consider the physician justified in going above the heads of the family, searching out the mother's sisters, and informing them of their risks and available options such as prenatal diagnosis? Do you believe that the physician acting in this way on behalf of the sisters, who may be at risk, can or should be sued for breach of confidentiality and trust for divulging private information? The obvious precedent for abridging the physician's duty of confidentiality may be found in statutes that require doctors to report persons with certain contagious diseases, such as meningitis. In such cases, these laws confer "absolute" immunity on the physician.

In an enlightened society, you would expect communication within families sufficient to ensure that children would be made aware of serious genetic disease in their own (possibly deceased) siblings or other close family members. Unfortunately, as stated earlier, it is not rare for parents to have hidden facts concerning an institutionalized or deceased defective child or close relative from their own children. Do you believe that such children (who may themselves be carriers of this genetic disease) have a legal right to be informed by their parents about disorders that affected their siblings or other family members? What legal recourse do these individuals have, and what is the physician's role in divulging their family history to them? The law is not especially helpful in this regard, but in many states a physician's license can be revoked for willfully betraying a professional secret. If you were engaged to be married and were worried about genetic disease affecting your future spouse because of family history, would you expect your spouse's physician to divulge that medical history to you? How would you feel if you were the one with the disease in your family, and your physician revealed it? And what about the ethics and legality of such action by the physician?

The Fetus

Questions, Questions

A veritable cascade of questions has enveloped all discussions concerning the fetus and the rights of parents. Who can dispute that parents have a right to have children? Does this right continue if they have a high risk of producing defective offspring? If the mother, for example, has a disease called phenylketonuria, she may damage 100 percent of her off-spring with virtually *all* of them being mentally retarded or having serious birth defects. There are those who argue that parents in such situations have no right to continue to pro-duce defective children. But does society, acting for the good of all, have the right or indeed the responsibility to adjudicate or even legislate for parents at risk for producing genetically abnormal offspring? Can society restrict the number of off-spring (as is now happening in India), or even offspring of a particular color? Does a group have any right to dictate on religious or metaphysical grounds that parents should not pre-vent the birth of a defective offspring? Can it be usefully ar-gued that the fetus is not merely a part of a woman's body, but a separate being over whom she may be presuming to exercise divine judgment? Then, if the fetus is indeed con-sidered to be a living being with equal rights, does not every fetus (or child) have the inalienable right to be born free of physical and mental defect? Does the fetus therefore have so-cietal rights, and if so, at what point during pregnancy?

The Fetus and the Law

Two major problems complicate all considerations of the legal status of the fetus. First, the fetus has been determined by the United States Supreme Court not to be a "person" as defined by the Constitution. Second, there remains a problem con-cerning when life begins. Certain religions are clear in their belief that life begins at conception. In efforts to define more specifically when life begins, medicine chose the concept of viability, defined as the ability to exist outside the womb. A fetus about 28 weeks along in pregnancy was, until recently, considered viable if able to exist on its own outside the mother's body. However, with increasing advances in tech-nology, the viability point has decreased to somewhere be-tween 24 and 28 weeks' gestation.

What is already abundantly clear is that the fetus does have legal rights. Many cases have been adjudicated, concluding each time that the fetus has property rights and may inherit.

Some courts have vested the fetus with legal rights as of conception, provided that it is subsequently *born alive* — even if only one gasp of breath is taken. Indeed, legal actions have been brought against individuals responsible for a father's death by children who were still in the mother's womb at the time. Other courts have recognized such fetal rights only if injury to the parent occurred at the time the fetus was in the "viable period."

The Tort of Wrongful Death

Injury to the fetus may be followed by spontaneous miscarriage, death in the womb, stillbirth, live birth followed by death, or live birth with injuries or defects. American courts have been inconsistent in allowing monetary awards for stillbirths and premature infants born alive but dying immediately or soon after birth. Some courts have ignored the stage of viability and made awards for injuries that occurred in the early weeks of pregnancy.

The Tort of Wrongful Life

More serious and difficult are the legal actions that might arise from what has been called the tort of "wrongful" life. A case brought before the Supreme Court of New Jersey is illustrative. The mother had testified she had informed her physicians that she had had German measles at two months of pregnancy. Both parents and the child brought a malpractice action against her physicians on the grounds that they had failed to inform her of possible congenital deformities, thereby preventing her from seeking an abortion. The child was indeed born with serious defects in sight, hearing, and speech. The court had to address the question whether, if the physicians had not been negligent, the child would not have been born at all! Or, is life with grave defects better than no life at all? The claim against the physician is, therefore, in essence, one for "wrongful" life. The New Jersey court disallowed the cause of action because the law did not recognize damages for allowing the birth of a child, even with defects.

In another case, pregnancy resulted following the rape of a mentally retarded woman by an inmate in the same state institution. Later, the child claimed that the state was negligent in allowing her conception. Again, the court ruled that there were strong policy and social reasons against providing such compensation.

"When" Is Life?

While the courts have already adjudicated cases concerning the legal rights of the fetus, society through its lawmakers has begun to debate and legislate. Nevertheless, neither the courts nor society will ever be able satisfactorily to settle the deep moral and ethical dilemmas that have beset the recent advances in prenatal diagnosis. Again and again it is asked: *when* does the fetus take on an individual existence? Is it at the moment of conception or perhaps when the fertilized egg implants in the wall of the womb? Is it at the moment the heartbeat is established or when brain wave activity is demonstrable? Or, is it only when the fetus is viable (between 24 to 28 weeks) and is able to exist outside the womb? While it will always be impossible to reconcile views of those who believe life begins at conception, or those who interpret life in terms of its quality, dignity, and humanness, it would seem reasonable to allow people to pursue their own beliefs without being forced to follow their religious, or other, dictates.

Human nature is such that if something good can be done, such as prenatal diagnosis, then it usually will be done. However, what you or I may call good and right someone else may call morally or ethically wrong. How, then, are guidelines established that reflect our humanistic concerns? Professor Joseph Fletcher, an acknowledged ethicist, now retired from the University of Virginia, believes "if human rights conflict with human needs, let needs prevail . . . rights are nothing but a formal recognition by society of certain human needs, and as needs change with changing conditions, so rights should change too."

Society

What may be good for you and your family may not necessarily be good for society as a whole. A *balance* of benefits is constantly being struck between individual needs and society's goals. The ability to prevent genetic disease by prenatal diagnosis has developed against the background of rapidly changing cultures all over the world. While in some countries, the specters of famine, disease, natural disasters, and war still loom large on the horizon, many other nations are caught up in their public concern for population growth, women's rights, the consequences of illegal or legal abortions, the number of *unwanted* children, the questions of euthanasia for the congenitally defective newborn and irreparably brain-damaged individuals, as well as the soaring costs of long-term medical care.

Historically, Western society has taken very definite steps to secure the best public health for the good of all. In the United States, many compulsory requirements have been issued by the individual states. There are numerous statutes in a variety of jurisdictions that require persons to be vaccinated or immunized against smallpox, measles, German measles, and poliomyelitis. A state requires testing for venereal disease and Rh (blood incompatibility) disease. A state may even demand treatment for venereal disease, tuberculosis, and for newborn eye infection (neonatal ophthalmia). A state may reserve the right to incarcerate those who are mentally incompetent. Most states prohibit all mating of persons as close as or closer than first cousins. Others currently have compulsory sterilization laws, and a significant number of jurisdictions retain legal authority to sterilize institutionalized mental defectives. A few states even permit the sterilization of certain convicted felons.

Detecting Carriers of Hereditary Disease

There has been a rash of state legislation governing the question of screening for carriers of hereditary disease. So hasty have some of these efforts been that in one state, Georgia, they inadvertently required the impossible — immunization for sickle cell anemia! To provide the largest number of options, it would be most sensible to provide young people at the time of marriage with tests to determine if they are carriers of certain genetic disorders. In this way, the best options are available to prevent the occurrence of any tragedies. Currently, the only test demanded at marriage is the one for venereal disease, such as syphilis. Wide-scale screening programs — especially for sickle cell anemia — have run into a variety of problems. It is to be expected, indeed should be demanded, that any information about a person's carrier status should be kept totally confidential. There have been a number of instances where the system of confidentiality has broken down, diminishing the utilization and value of such programs. One aspect of this breach of privacy has particular implications for the carrier individual. For example, if a life insurance company has the information, it may refuse to provide insurance or at least step up the premiums. While for the vast majority of disorders, individuals who carry certain diseases are not at any additional risk themselves, there are occasional examples where this is not in fact the case, so that some carriers may ultimately be shown to have a diminished life expectancy.

Costs and Benefits in Prenatal Diagnosis

You may feel that it is futile to consider the benefits of preventive programs when treatment is not yet available and abortion is the only viable option. Some facts are however unsuppressible. The already over-burdened taxpayer often feels that where prevention is possible, it should be pursued. The burgeoning health care costs of institutionalization for the defective individual represents a clear chronic financial drain. It is known that the projected lifetime care in an institution for one child with Down's syndrome is at least a quarter of a million dollars. The estimate for lifetime care of spina bifida children is between $100,000 to $250,000. The taxpayer is understandably concerned. Each year in the United States, close to 20,000 children are born with some kind of chromosomal abnormality and about 8000 with anencephaly or spina bifida (see Chapter 9), to mention the two most common birth defects. Institutional care costs are presently about $6000 per year. *Society*, therefore, makes a commitment each year in excess of 2 billion dollars for only two birth defects. The commitment by society over 20 years at current costs (which of course will not apply) will have grown to over 40 billion dollars!

Hence, willingly or not, we are forced to consider the economic aspects of prenatal diagnosis, remembering that these techniques are mainly applied to disorders with irreparable mental defect or fatal or serious genetic disease. Taking into consideration the cost of amniocentesis and prenatal studies, as well as the cost of elective abortion, estimates have been made of total "prevention" costs. If one considers only women who are thirty-five years and over in the United States alone, then the necessary costs, provided all such women had the test, approach 63 million dollars. As we have said, mothers thirty-five years and over, while constituting only 5 percent of the childbearing population, give birth to about 25 percent of all children with Down's syndrome. Projections for the cost of lifetime care for defective offspring born to mothers aged thirty-five years and over show that society would be committing about 2 billion dollars in one year — about 32 times the cost of prevention through prenatal diagnosis and elective abortion.

Law and Prenatal Studies

During the mid-seventies, there has been an extremely poor utilization of prenatal studies that are available in the United States. It is conceivable that legislative support will ultimately be seen as a necessity for an effective program. Should such an eventuality come to pass, the problem would be to distinguish between voluntary and mandatory prenatal diagnosis and voluntary and mandatory selective abortion of defective fetuses. A voluntary program of amniocentesis followed by voluntary abortion of genetically defective fetuses would appear to be the most equitable, and least offensive, to

religious and other groups. Any program that makes amniocentesis mandatory is likely to be equally firm about abortion
of defective fetuses. Since compulsory sterilization statutes
do exist in at least 21 states, society has already established
the power to prevent the conception of potentially defective
offspring. Attempts at such legislation, as stated in this chapter, were made more possible after the United States Supreme
Court ruling on abortion. But I believe we can nevertheless
rest assured that any statute aimed at mandatory amniocentesis and compulsory abortion is likely to fail in view of its
assault on the rights to procreational privacy and on those
rights prohibiting unreasonable searches and seizures.

It would seem wisest for legislators and government to ex-
pend their efforts at educating the people about the recent
advances in medicine, and in this context, appropriating
funds aimed at the prevention of genetic disease. Should society see fit to introduce legislation concerning prenatal diagnosis, I hope that its essential thrust would be to assist the
further development of technology and its easy accessibility to
those who need it most. Any such legislation must be noncoercive and nondiscriminatory, paying special heed to the
respect for the freedom of expression and rights of the individual. At the same time, each of us should remain acutely
aware of those tragedies "we daily see [that are] but hadn't
ought to be."

CHAPTER 18

Heart Disease, Hypertension, and Heredity

WILL YOU HAVE A HEART ATTACK? Why? When? Does it matter if you do or do not have a family history of heart disease? What can you do about heart disease?

Diseases of the heart and blood vessels affect virtually everyone. Both hereditary and environmental factors acting separately or, more commonly, together cause the vast majority of these disorders. I will focus on the hereditary aspects of diseases of the heart and blood vessels, drawing attention only when necessary to environmental influences that may interact with hereditary predisposition.

Hereditary disorders of the heart and blood vessels may take on many different forms, three of which are of special importance. First, you or your child may have been born with a structural defect of the heart, such as a hole-in-the-heart or a narrowed valve. Second, in your middle years of life you may have or may develop coronary artery disease, a disease of the main blood vessels supplying the heart, or develop high blood pressure. Third, heart disease occurs in association with different types of hereditary disorders. Let us consider these three major categories of hereditary heart disease separately and in some detail.

Birth Defects of the Heart

The heart is formed during the first eight weeks of pregnancy. Hence it is not unusual for a prospective mother, not even knowing that she is pregnant, to have already completed eight weeks of pregnancy and be carrying a fetus whose heart is already formed. She may unwittingly have been taking certain drugs or been exposed to certain infections that could cause birth defects of the heart. Heart defects due to German measles may include a hole between the two lower chambers or ventricles of the heart, called ventricular septal defect; or a too narrow valve outlet of the pulmonary artery to the lung, called pulmonary stenosis; or the persistence of a communication between the aorta, the large blood vessel that leaves the heart to supply the rest of the body, and the large pulmonary artery that supplies the lung — a disorder called patent ductus arteriosus.

It is known that virtually all these structural abnormalities of the heart, such as communicating holes between chambers or narrow valves, can also arise through hereditary mechanisms. Frequently, however, it is virtually impossible to separate out those cases where the cause has been environmental rather than hereditary. Indeed, interaction between both these causes is the most common explanation for their occurrence. Some of these heart defects, for example, occur more frequently in births during the fall and winter, suggesting the action of an environmental factor such as a virus (see chapters 5 and 9).

When it is clearly difficult to separate out environmental from hereditary factors, it might seem safer to *assume* a hereditary factor with risks for recurrence of 3 to 5 percent; if a couple has had two children affected, the risks for recurrence rise to 8 to 12 percent; and if three are affected, the recurrence risks approximate 25 percent. If one of the parents is affected by one of these heart disorders, then the risk in a first pregnancy may be 3 to 5 percent of having a child with a similar disorder. The heart defects that fall into these risk categories include the aforementioned hole between the two lower chambers of the heart, a hole between the upper chambers of the heart called atrial septal defect, patent ductus arteriosus, and pulmonary stenosis, to name only the major types.

Diseases of the Heart and Blood Vessels

The most common cause of death by far in the United States and probably in most Western industrialized societies is disease of the heart and blood vessels. The vast majority of these diseases are due to thinning and hardening of the walls of arteries, called arteriosclerosis. The most important type of arteriosclerosis is called atherosclerosis, which by itself is the greatest single cause of death in the United States.

Atherosclerosis

This is not a new disease, although it has become a major scourge of modern civilization. It has been recognized in Egyptian mummies and even described in the ancient writings of the Greeks. In atherosclerosis, fatty and fibrous substances are deposited and form streaks, patches, and nodules mainly on the inner walls of the largest arteries, including the three coronary arteries that supply the heart. These fatty and fibrous substances increase in size, become associated with blood clots, and eventually can obstruct a coronary artery to cause a heart attack. Evidence that atherosclerosis begins in childhood is clear. Children dying before puberty have been found with patches of it in their major arteries. Indeed, United States soldiers dying in battle in the Korean War, less than twenty years of age, frequently had well-established atherosclerosis.

The heart attack basically results from a lack of blood (and therefore oxygen) reaching the heart muscle. Such heart attacks are the main cause of death in males after thirty-five years of age and in all persons over age forty-five. Deaths before fifty occur predominantly in men, and about one-third of all deaths from these heart attacks in males occur before age sixty-five. Between thirty-five to fifty-five years of age, the death rate is five times higher in white men as opposed to white women in the United States. This difference becomes less significant after the menopause. Women with high blood pressure, diabetes, or an early menopause share the same risks as the male. The six nations that have the highest death rates for white men between forty-five and sixty-four years of age are South Africa, the United States, England, Scotland, Canada, and Australia. Death rates in these age brackets are much lower in most Western European countries and Latin America.

In Japan, the death rates in this age group are about one-fifth of those in the United States.

Other factors producing variation are socioeconomical: the higher the income, the better the standard of living, and the more frequent the occurrence of premature heart attacks. Elements that might bring on more attacks among the affluent groups are the higher fat content of the diet and the decreased amount of physical work. Generally, however, significant differences in the frequency of heart attacks among different cultures are not easily explained. For example, Scots and North Americans have a death rate from premature heart attacks more than twice that of Swedes. While premature heart disease is decidedly common among the whites of South Africa, it is extremely unusual in blacks living in the same locality. Differences in the occurrence of heart disease associated with high blood fat levels (cholesterol or triglycerides) between different groups in the same country, or between national groups, probably reflect a fundamental variation in hereditary susceptibility to the particular environmental factors operative in different cultures.

Factors That Cause, Aggravate, or Precipitate Heart Attacks

Notwithstanding the possibility of genetic predisposition, other recognized factors are known either to cause, aggravate, or precipitate premature heart attacks. Whether you are genetically predisposed or not, attention to the following hazards may help you prevent premature heart disease:

1. High blood fat (cholesterol or triglycerides) levels caused by a variety of factors
2. High blood pressure
3. Cigarette smoking
4. Sugar diabetes
5. Lack of physical exercise
6. Obesity
7. Emotional stress

8. Family history of premature heart attacks in near relatives, especially parents or brothers or sisters
9. Oral contraceptives

Women under forty years of age taking oral contraceptives have a negligible risk of coronary heart disease, provided they have none of the risk factors just mentioned. In particular, oral contraceptives should be used with great caution (or perhaps better, not at all) in women over forty years of age, those with a family history of coronary heart disease, and those who smoke more than 20 cigarettes a day.

Women taking oral contraceptives have also been shown to have increased blood fat levels and to have an associated increase in risk of disease of the blood vessels supplying the brain. This would mean clotting within those blood vessels and lead to strokes. Certainly the evidence suggests that heart attacks in women before the menopause occur more frequently among those taking oral contraceptives. It is not yet clear whether women after menopause increase their risk of heart attack by using female hormones. Men who smoke more than one pack of cigarettes a day have 70 percent more heart attacks than nonsmoking males. The increase in the death rate is clearly proportional to the amount smoked. The relation between smoking and premature heart attacks also applies to women, but not as severely as to men.

Hereditary High Risk
Coronary Heart Disease

Studies have shown that between 50 to 85 percent of all individuals contracting coronary heart disease before they are fifty have high blood cholesterol levels and/or high blood fat triglyceride levels. There are four hereditary disorders that can almost invariably be found responsible for this condition.

Familial Hypercholesterolemia

In this very common disorder, high blood cholesterol levels are associated with coronary artery disease. It is one of the most widespread of all genetic diseases that afflict people! Approximately 1 in every 500 of the population possesses the gene, making familial hypercholesterolemia even more prevalent than cystic fibrosis or sickle cell anemia.

Familial hypercholesterolemia is transmitted through families via a dominant form of inheritance (see Chapter 5). This means that if you are affected, there would be a 50 percent chance that each of your children will develop the same disorder. Should it happen that both you and your spouse carry the same abnormal (mutant) gene for familial hypercholesterolemia, the risk of having an affected child rises to 75 percent in each pregnancy. Those children who receive the gene from both you and your spouse will be severely affected. Their blood cholesterol levels will be so high, because of the double dose of the abnormal gene, that they will show fatty accumulations that can be seen on the skin (around the eyes or tendons) and, moreover, they will develop coronary artery disease and have heart attacks in adolescence or even earlier. The children who have received an abnormal gene for familial hypercholesterolemia from each parent have not thus far been known to survive beyond thirty years of age.

Familial hypercholesterolemia may be detected at birth by analyzing blood samples from the umbilical cord, and of course from blood samples taken later in childhood. You should note that a single "normal" cholesterol level does not simply rule out the possibility that you may have the disorder, especially if you are at risk, since some overlap of cholesterol values do occur between those affected and normal family members. If you really are at risk, then in addition to repeating blood samples for cholesterol estimation, it would be important to test for cholesterol in a more sophisticated way (determination of cholesterol in low-density lipoprotein). Remember always that the blood cholesterol testing should be done after an overnight fast if the result is to be reliable.

About 50 percent of affected males with this disorder will usually have some kind of symptoms of coronary artery disease by the age of fifty or, at least, sixty years. The risk of coronary artery disease for women carrying the genes is somewhat lower than males but is nevertheless greater than that of the general female population. Between 3 and 6 percent of middle-aged survivors of heart attacks in the United States, England, and Finland have familial hypercholesterolemia.

The available treatment includes reduction of cholesterol in the diet and of saturated fat intake. Certain drugs like cholestyramine resin may be used for treatment to further decrease the blood cholesterol by as much as 30 percent. The unfortunate person who has received the abnormal gene from both affected parents requires drastic measures that include major surgical shunting of blood, or exchange plasma transfusions, and other procedures not free of danger themselves.

Recently, cells grown from the skin (cultured fibroblasts) have been shown to manifest the presence of the abnormal gene for familial hypercholesterolemia. Hence, it has become possible to make the prenatal diagnosis of this disorder early in fetal life. In the rare situation where both parents know they have the gene, they may select the option to terminate a pregnancy when the fetus can be shown to have the severest form of the disease, which will cause heart attacks and death by adolescence or earlier.

Familial Hypertriglyceridemia

This hereditary disorder is almost twice as common as familial hypercholesterolemia just discussed above! Its frequency in the population has been estimated at close to 1 in 300 people. It is also associated with premature coronary artery disease but appreciably less so than in familial hypercholesterolemia. As opposed to the latter condition, this disorder is characterized by high levels of triglycerides or blood fats and is *not* usually associated with high blood cholesterol levels.

From the available evidence, it seems that it is also transmitted as a dominant trait, that is, if you have the disorder there should be a 50 percent chance that each of your children will have the same problem. In actuality, and despite what was theoretically expected, only about 10 to 20 percent of children and adolescents of such affected parents appear to show signs of it.

For reasons that are not yet clear, diabetes, resistance to

insulin, and obesity seem to occur more frequently in individuals with high blood triglyceride levels. Very high blood fat levels are found especially in persons with this disorder when their diabetes has gone untreated, or after excessive alcohol intake, as well as after taking oral contraceptives or estrogen hormones. Obviously, then, if you are affected by such a disorder, diabetes should be watched for, and excess alcohol and the use of female hormones should be avoided. In addition, if there is obesity, weight reduction is very important. The drug Atromid-S (clofibrate) has been used with the intention of lowering the blood fat levels in this condition.

Familial Combined Hyperlipidemia

This third type of hereditary high blood fat disorder is even more common than either the first or second type just described, affecting close to 1 in 200 of the population. Again, in this disorder, there is a close association with a high frequency of heart attacks. The disorder may not become apparent until a person is in his or her late twenties. In about one-third of cases, both the blood cholesterol and blood fat or triglyceride levels are raised; roughly another third has only high blood cholesterol, with the last third showing only high blood fat levels.

Again, the hereditary transmission here is by a dominant trait: if you have it there is a 50 percent chance you will pass it on to each of your children. Treatment similar to that given the other high blood fat disorders is usually recommended.

At least one of the three hereditary disorders just discussed affects 1 in every 100 individuals in the United States, and probably in other Western nations. The enormity of this figure needs no embellishment. Heart attacks kill a large number of people in whom one of these disorders has never been recognized. Specific diagnosis is not simple, as family history analysis and other studies may be necessary to differentiate the three diseases described above from a fourth type of blood disorder called polygenic hypercholesterolemia.

Polygenic Hypercholesterolemia

This is not an easily defined disorder since, as the name implies, the high blood cholesterol is in this case due to the interaction of genes and environmental factors. About 50 percent of all Americans under thirty years of age have elevated blood cholesterol levels. The percentage is even higher from forty years of age and on. In this condition, the triglycerides are not elevated. It would therefore be wise for all adults in our country to have a periodic check of their blood cholesterol. The approach to prevention and treatment is the same as discussed for the first three disorders.

Familial but Not Genetic

There are many studies that document coronary heart disease aggregates in families. These studies are, however, difficult to interpret, since no division was made into the types of diseases we have just discussed. Moreover, they have generally also not separated out environmental effects, such as smoking or dietary habits, common to family members, which are acquired rather than inherited.

There are some other confounding factors that are sporadic and secondary. Cases occur, for instance, of high blood cholesterol levels found without any family history of heart disease; these may simply be sporadic or due to other secondary causes such as hypothyroidism and a type of kidney disease. Not rarely, sporadic cases are found where the blood fats are elevated — again without a family history of heart disease — and called sporadic hypertriglyceridemia.

Heart Disease and Stress

The nine risk factors for heart disease mentioned earlier make it clear to you that all that is familial is not necessarily hereditary. One other example is too good to omit. The Swedes studied *identical* twins, only one of whom had coronary heart disease. They focused on the psychological aspects in the lives of the twins. Their observations showed that the higher the degree of dissatisfaction with life, the greater was the severity of coronary heart disease.

It's the Blood Groups Again!

We mentioned earlier (Chapter 6) the HLA (histocompatibility antigens) blood group system. Australian researchers have suggested that the blood group HLA-8 (and possibly W15) may be linked to genes that predispose to high blood cholesterol and subsequent coronary heart disease. Certainly the individual with the HLA-8 blood group appears to have a much greater risk of developing diabetes in childhood, overactive thyroid glands, and other disorders. Hence, notwithstanding any dietary indiscretions or smoking, your HLA blood group may influence your chances for developing coronary heart disease.

The Coronary Artery Blueprint

By now, you will not be surprised to hear that even the anatomy — the layout — of the three main coronary arteries and their interconnections is probably genetically determined. Particular differences in the way the heart muscle is supplied by blood may, on occasion, make certain areas more vulnerable to the effects of increasing blockage, by atherosclerosis, of the coronary arteries. Moreover, genetic influences affect the actual construction of the coronary arteries themselves. For example, Ashkenazic Jews in Israel, who have a higher prevalence of coronary artery disease than Yemenite Jews or Bedouins in Israel, have a greater development of the inner lining (intima) and muscle-elastic layer of the coronary arteries than the other two groups. These structural features may enhance the formation and/or deposition of cholesterol, that is, the process of atherosclerosis.

Other hereditary high blood fat disorders do occur, but are very rare. The risks may vary from 25 to 50 percent for each child having the disease if one or both parents are affected.

Premature coronary heart disease occurring before fifty years of age may again be a prominent feature.

What Should You Do?

If you already know that you are affected by one of these hereditary high blood fat diseases, then one would hope that you have already stopped smoking and are on a schedule of treatment, including weight reduction, careful control of diabetes, exclusion of oral contraceptives, estrogen hormones, and alcohol. The additional drugs mentioned above or others recommended by your physician may also be helpful.

It is more likely that as you read this section, you may not be aware whether you are in fact affected or not. If you have, or had, a parent, a brother, or a sister who had a heart attack before fifty years of age, then you would be advised to have a general checkup and request fasting blood cholesterol and triglyceride studies. Treatment is available, and you would be doing yourself and your family harm by not taking adequate care of yourself. The United States Coronary Drug Project did show, however, that drug treatment to reduce blood fats was of much less importance than dietary modification and attention to the high risk factors mentioned earlier. Incidentally, the blood cholesterol and fat tests may need to be repeated two or three times, especially if there is reason to suspect one of these disorders. Other family members who have not yet reached thirty years of age should also be re-tested later, since children and adolescents frequently may not show the characteristic high blood cholesterol or fat levels.

To Screen or Not to Screen

Knowing how serious an impact heart disease has on all of us, due consideration has been given to testing blood samples early in life. The idea, of course, is that early diagnosis would lead to the instigation of preventive measures. Consequently, tests have been run on blood collected from the baby's cord right at birth, while other studies have focused on blood samples taken during the first year of life. Neither approach has really succeeded, mainly because the predictive value of a high or even a normal blood cholesterol (or triglyceride) has been unsatisfactory. For example, some children *without* a family history of heart attacks have been found with high blood cholesterol levels at birth. Others have had normal cholesterol values at birth and been found to have the genetic condition at one year of age. Finally, genetic disorders with high blood fat levels may not manifest themselves until adolescence or later.

At present, instead of screening every child born, it would seem wisest to examine samples only from the children of a parent with one of the first three genetic disorders with high blood cholesterol and/or triglycerides that we have just considered.

Hypertension

The Problem

Hypertension affects about 24 million adults in the United States and figures prominently as a cause of early death and of chronic illness through its main complications of strokes and heart and kidney failure. The higher the blood pressure, the greater the risk of these eventualities. Treatment is recognized as being effective and is especially helpful in about 30 percent of those individuals with moderate to severe high blood pressure. Treatment in such cases is certainly worthwhile. When there is only mild hypertension, the efficacy of treatment is more uncertain. Only about 15 to 20 percent of people with hypertension in the United States receive full treatment at present. The main problem is that most people do not have their blood pressure checked and are not aware that they are hypertensive. This may also be the reason why the early onset of hypertension has been overlooked for so long. (When did you last have your blood pressure checked?)

The Causes of High Blood Pressure

The actual cause of hypertension is recognized in only about 10 percent of all cases. The most common known causes are kidney disease or disease or disorder of the blood vessels supplying the kidney. Only in a few percent of the recognized causes of high blood pressure are there opportunities through surgery to correct the defect and cure the hypertension.

It has increasingly been recognized recently that women using oral contraceptives have between a two to six times greater likelihood of developing hypertension than nonusers. If you are taking oral contraceptives and have been found to have high blood pressure, it would be wiser to consult with your physician and perhaps to discontinue such medications for at least six months in order to assess the impact of these pills on your blood pressure.

Hereditary Aspects

While the cause of hypertension remains undiscovered about 90 percent of the time, there is a great deal of evidence pointing to hereditary elements. Although it is well recognized that hypertension tends to aggregate within families, it is not at all clear how it is transmitted from parent to child. It is, however, likely that some of the mechanisms that may ultimately lead to high blood pressure are governed by hereditary factors.

You might think that a simple in-depth investigation of all the blood pressures within a family repeated over a period of years might answer the question. This is unfortunately not the case. Screening out environmental influences can be extremely difficult. Consider the study done recently in the west of Scotland, where heart disease is very common.

It had been established in other studies that hypertension and heart disease occurred commonly in areas with soft-drinking water supplies. In the west of Scotland (and elsewhere), not only is the drinking water extremely soft, but it is frequently tapped and stored in lead plumbing systems. The acidic nature of soft water facilitates the entry of the lead into drinking water. The Scottish researchers, not surprisingly, found that hypertension in that area was associated with high lead levels in the blood. Whether this is pure chance and not a cause and effect relationship is still uncertain. Nevertheless it is bothersome, since at least two other studies point to the same association between increased blood lead levels and hypertension.

It is known that high blood pressure is more common among blacks at all ages, of both sexes, than among whites. (High blood pressure among the Japanese is also very common.) About one in four blacks ultimately develops hypertension. While this observation may clearly implicate genetic mechanisms, it is also effectively argued that blacks have different cooking habits than whites. In particular, they are known to consume more salt than whites do. Salt, of course, is known to aggravate hypertension. The matter becomes more complicated when you recognize that calcium in the diet, especially milk and milk products, may act to dampen the effect of salt on the blood pressure. It is a fact that many more blacks than whites are intolerant to milk — actually, to a sugar in milk called lactose, and this intolerance is genetically determined. Hence it has been argued, in a rather circuitous way, that there are hereditary factors that influence the blood pressure of blacks. Many others undoubtedly exist.

Laboratory animals have been used to estimate the relative importance of heredity in development of hypertension. Two inbred strains of rats were produced with similar blood pressures. A strikingly dissimilar response to salt intake occurred in these two strains, the one hardly reacting, while the other produced severely high blood pressure and died from kidney failure in weeks. Hence, some hereditary influence was implied in this experiment. But such factors in humans, I repeat, may be those that interact with, or even depend on, elements in the environment.

High blood pressure is frequently associated with a number of rare genetic disorders, such as polycystic kidney disease and also Fabry's disease. Here the hypertension is a feature or complication of illnesses with a definite hereditary pattern.

In sum, therefore, your chance of developing high blood pressure depends on largely unknown hereditary factors, whether you are white or black and what your family history has been. A group of hereditary disorders — including some cases of hypertension — are probably transmitted from parent to child via a multifactor mechanism called polygenic inheritance. If one of your parents had, for no known cause, severe hypertension, then your risk of high blood pressure might be 3 to 5 percent. But it is far too early still to provide reliable risk figures when so much is yet to be understood about the genetics of hypertension. It would seem safer, if it is in your family history, or if you are black, to be certain that your blood pressure is checked at least yearly, to avoid being overweight, to avoid oral contraceptives and smoking, and to cut down on salt.

Heart disease can be a depressing subject since so many of us will eventually succumb to it. If we have lived at least our three score and ten years, it is not as tragic as being cut off in the prime of our lives. About 16 million people in the United States alone, simply on the basis of a genetic condition or predisposition leading to elevated blood cholesterol, are presently at risk for having a heart attack before fifty-five years of age. Are you 1 of the 7 in every 100 in this category?

Remember that in heart disease, as in so many other things, prevention is much more effective than treatment.

CHAPTER 19

Heredity and Cancer

IT IS WELL RECOGNIZED that cancer tends to aggregate in families. There is no longer any doubt that susceptibility to cancer is inherited. The question is, rather, how do your genes predispose you to cancer and how may such harmful genes be identified in each of us? For the majority of cancer cases, the pattern of inheritance has not generally been along the classic lines — dominant, recessive, sex-linked — that we discussed in Chapter 5. Some specific types of cancer are, however, transmitted in predictable hereditary patterns, and we will discuss these in some detail later in this chapter.

But What Is Cancer?

Before we go further, it should be understood that a cancer is a group of cells, probably originating from one cell, that begins to grow abnormally, invades the surrounding tissues, and spreads through the blood stream and the lymphatic system to other parts of the body. It is then deemed a malignant tumor. If a tumor simply grows and remains in its tissue of origin without spreading, it is called benign and can be easily removed, leaving the person with no risk of recurrence. The distinguishing feature of a malignant tumor is therefore not so much the abnormal growth of certain cells, but rather a defect in the body mechanisms that normally set the territorial limits of cells and keep the abnormally growing cells from invading other tissues or spreading to other parts of the body.

While cancers may arise in any single tissue of the body, broadly speaking there are mainly three recognized types. The first are called *carcinomas*: they arise in sheets of cells that cover the outside skin of the body as well as line the inside of all hollow organs, such as the stomach. Second, there are those that arise in the blood-forming cells of bone marrow, lymph glands, or spleen — and these are called *leukemias* or *lymphomas*. The third and rarest type of cancer originates in the bones and connective tissues of the body and is called a *sarcoma*.

The Magnitude of the Problem

The probability that any of us will develop cancer at some time during our lifetime is about 1 in 4. The estimated total of new cases of cancer occurring at all body sites in 1976 approximated 675,000 cases in the United States alone. Not surprisingly, after heart disease, cancer is the second most common cause of death in the United States.

Cancer develops most frequently in association with aging, and this applies to all its varieties. It is known that the death rate from cancer of the large intestine increases about 1000 times between the ages of twenty and eighty years, and most of this increase occurs after age sixty.

About half of all cancer deaths are caused by cancers of three organs: the lungs, the large intestine, and the breast. Trying to determine the frequency of a cancer can be quite difficult. For example, the usual estimate of cancer of the prostate in seventy-year-old men is about 200 cases per 100,000 men per year (0.2 percent). However, examination of the prostate glands at autopsies of seventy-year-old men who have died from other causes have shown cancer that is still microscopic in size in 15 to 20 percent of these cases. The incidence of prostatic cancer measured by this technique would therefore be 100 times greater than that observed in patients who have symptoms. Hence, it is possible that each of us may develop several groups of abnormally growing cells in various tissues. The crucial point is that we do not know what factors would allow those abnormal cells to spread through tissues and lead to clinically obvious cancer. The one thing that is certain is that more easily observed tissues allow more careful surveillance. The stomach, for example, is harder to examine than the skin. In fact, a recent survey in a rural district of Tennessee revealed that about 4 percent of the adult population had some kind of skin cancer. Obviously, the better the surveillance, the quicker the diagnosis, the more likely the cure.

Genetics or Environment?

Cancer in Twins

One of the classic methods of determining the role of heredity in disease has been the examination of identical and non-identical twins. Identical twins arise from a single fertilized egg or ovum and should then have the same tendency to develop any disease that is influenced by hereditary factors. If a disease is genetic, there should, of course, be a higher rate of concordance in identical versus nonidentical twins. Observations for cancer of the breast, stomach, intestine, and for leukemia suggest a rate for identical twins double that for nonidentical twins, which simply supports the evidence that hereditary factors are clearly operating — at least in these cancers. It was also observed, especially in Japanese studies, that the parents of children with leukemia are more frequently related than are the parents of children without leukemia. There appears, furthermore, to be an increased susceptibility in the siblings of a child with cancer. Brothers and sisters of children with brain tumors may have as much as a tenfold chance of dying from tumors of the brain, bones, or soft tissues. Careful *lifetime* medical surveillance of such persons is obviously important.

We have been talking about the rarer cases. Mostly, cancer seems to reflect the interaction between genes and environmental agents, such as the correlation between lung cancer and cigarettes.

The Immigrants

Cancer occurring in a few individuals in the same family living in the same state or country immediately raises a very complex question. Is heredity or environment at work here? There are a few clues provided by groups emigrating from one country to another. Take, for example, the incidence of cancer of the stomach in Japan, much more common there than in the United States. (In contrast, cancer of the large intestine, the breast, and the prostate are much less common in Japan than in the United States.) It has been noted that when Japanese emigrate to the United States, these differences in the incidence of cancer are lost within a generation or two. Since, for the most part, Japanese immigrants and their children have tended to marry within their ethnic group, the change in incidence of cancer is probably more related to their changed environment than to genetic factors.

Another example is the Jews who emigrated to Israel from Europe or the United States. They have been found to have an incidence of cancer more typical of the country from which they originated. Their children born in Israel, however, were found to have a much lower incidence of almost all kinds of cancer, similar to the Jewish population already in the area. Since families are likely to stay in the same areas, or at least in the same countries, it is difficult to separate out the factors. The problem is further bedeviled by the likelihood that certain environmental agents may have initiated the cancer mechanism a few decades before the patient actually comes to the doctor with an obvious tumor. The frequency of lung cancer is directly proportional not to the number of cigarettes smoked this year but rather to the number the patient smoked about 20 years ago! In a similar way, cancers occurring as a result of exposure to certain industrial chemicals may take 10 to 20 years or more to appear — the victim already being in retirement. One curious example of the long "incubation" period, which can be so deceptive, is cancer of the penis. This cancer is mainly seen in old men. However, it is now well established that cancers of the penis can be prevented by circumcision in the *first few days* of life but not if circumcision is delayed for a few years.

Genes and Cancer

The most reasonable theory that explains the clustering of cancer in old age proposes that each cell has several genes that either separately or together restrain it from growing abnormally, that is, becoming a cancer. Since genes may undergo mutation either spontaneously or because of environmental agents, such a likelihood increases with increasing age of the cell. Perhaps after as few as five mutations, the restraints on a cell are no longer effective, and the abnormal growth and spread begin. The implication of this theory is that many cancers are likely to be the end result of a number of mutations, some of which probably began quite early in the person's life. Such mutations may have been initiated by environmental agents acting on the embryo or fetus in the womb. The diethylstilbestrol (DES) question is the best example.

The DES Disaster

A report in 1971 from Professor Arthur L. Herbst and colleagues at the Massachusetts General Hospital drew attention for the first time to the occurrence of cancer of the female genital tract, mainly the vagina, in the daughters of mothers who took a sex hormone called diethylstilbestrol during early pregnancy. They observed seven cases of vaginal cancer occurring in females under the age of twenty-two years. Cancer of the vagina in this age group is extraordinarily rare. By August 1973, 170 patients had been studied, 100 of whom had vaginal cancer while 70 had cancer of the cervix. The total dosages of DES ingested by their mothers throughout pregnancy varied markedly. For most cases, it appeared that treatment had begun prior to the eighteenth week of pregnancy, suggesting exposure during the time when the female genital tract was being formed.

The Massachusetts General Hospital group continued their studies by examining as many daughters as possible of mothers who had taken DES during pregnancy. In these prospective studies, they found 110 exposed daughters and compared them to 82 who had not been exposed. Among the former, there were striking changes in the genital tract of both the vagina and cervix. All the changes were benign. They did notice, however, that abnormal-looking cells in the cervix occurred in virtually all this group but in only half of those not exposed to DES in the womb.

Some efforts were made to estimate the number of girls in the United States whose mothers had taken DES or similar hormones during pregnancy. Estimates were made using the data from the Boston Collaborative Drug Surveillance Program indicating that from 1960 to 1970, in the United States, 100,000 to 160,000 females were born who had been exposed to these hormones while in their mothers' wombs. No estimates were available in the late 1940s and 1950s when these drugs were probably more commonly used for the treatment of high risk pregnancy. It appears likely that the exposed female population in the United States numbers in the hundreds of thousands and possibly even in the millions. For these women, the risk of malignancy developing is still uncertain and has been estimated to be less than 4 in 1000 under the age of twenty-five years. On the average, these cancers appear at about seventeen and a half years of age, with over 90 percent of the females involved being over the age of twelve.

While the exact mechanism that ultimately leads to the formation of cancer in the female genital tract is unknown, it appears that a whole spectrum of changes varying from the benign to the malignant occurs. Hence, it is absolutely crucial for any woman exposed to DES before birth to be examined by her gynecologist at least once or twice a year for the rest of her life. Remember, cancer is curable if diagnosed early enough.

Other Delayed Consequences of Exposure in the Womb

In addition to DES, there are other known and probably mostly unknown hazards from exposing the embryo or fetus during pregnancy. For example, exposing the fetus to x-rays during diagnostic studies of the mother has been reported in some studies to be associated with an increase in the risk of childhood cancer, especially leukemia, years later. Indeed, one study suggested an increase of 40 percent in the risk of cancer, including leukemia, in children who had been exposed to x-rays while in the womb. Not unexpectedly, some studies have shown that the risk of childhood cancer increased with larger doses of x-rays as well as with earlier exposures during pregnancy. While it is true that other elements may be important in the development of cancer following x-rays, such as individual susceptibility, there is sufficient evidence for women to avoid unnecessary x-ray examinations during pregnancy.

Almost 20 years ago, the observation was made suggesting an association between viral infection of the mother during pregnancy and the development of cancer in the child born subsequently. One retrospective study analyzed records of women who developed chicken pox or mumps at any stage of pregnancy, or German measles in the first 18 weeks. While no children died from leukemia as a result of German measles or mumps, a significant number of leukemia deaths in children were reported by the mothers who had had chicken pox in pregnancy. The available evidence must be viewed as inconclusive, through there are serious suspicions linking viral infection in a pregnant mother not only with leukemia, but also with other cancers in her offspring.

Cigarette Smoking

The relation of smoking to lung cancer is another example of the cooperation of a gene with the environment to wreak havoc on the human body. You will have noticed individuals who have smoked heavily all their lives without developing lung cancer, though in all probability they have chronic bronchitis and emphysema. From accumulated data, we find that certain individuals have a predisposition to develop lung cancer, smoking inducing in them the activity of a certain enzyme, called arylhydrocarbonhydroxylase, which reacts with compounds in cigarette smoke and in turn causes the cancer. This enzyme is of course under the control of a specific gene. One goal of genetic work in progress is to determine, if possible, which individuals are especially susceptible to cancer from smoking.

Other Agents

While cigarette smoking is the most well known factor because of the high incidence of lung cancer, there are many other environmental agents that alone or by interacting with a genetic predisposition may cause cancer. X-ray exposure can cause leukemia; alcohol is implicated in producing cancer of the liver; many different industrial toxins affect various organs, as do some drugs and hormones, certain viruses, possibly some food additives or preservatives. Too much sunlight can cause skin cancer. A number of agents may not necessarily cause cancer directly, but may enhance the likelihood of its occurrence, as in the case for cancer of the uterus, linked to the use of the hormone estrogen.

Breast Cancer and Heredity

One of the most common cancers — that of the breast — is known to occur two or three times more frequently in close relatives of affected persons. Currently, it appears that there are at least two main types of breast cancer, one occurring before the menopause and one after menopause. Undoubtedly, other types also occur. Available evidence indicates that women with cancer occurring before the menopause have affected relatives (grandmother, mother, aunt, or sister) in 6 to 8 percent of cases, in contrast to no increase in the frequency of breast cancer in the relatives of women having the disease after the menopause. When cancer has been found in both breasts, the frequency in relatives of the patient increased to 13 percent. If the woman was both premenopausal and had cancer in both breasts, then the frequency in relatives rose to 17 percent, in contrast to the frequency in relatives of women with cancer in one breast only — a figure of 3.4 percent. The frequency of cancer in both breasts is about 10 percent in all women with family histories and about 15 percent in those who were diagnosed before the menopause. Clearly, then, hereditary factors play an important role in women with early onset (ages twenty to forty-nine years), especially in both breasts, compared to those with late-onset breast cancer and only a single tumor. But note that only 3 percent of all breast cancers occur via a recognized hereditary mechanism.

In those families with women having cancer in both breasts occurring before the menopause, a dominant form of inheritance has been suggested. The direct implication would then be that a female whose mother had bilateral breast cancer *may* have a risk as high as 50 percent of developing a similar cancer. It would seem judicious for such women not only to have careful breast examination and mammography yearly, but also to become expert at palpation of their own breasts.

There appears to be at least another hereditary subtype of breast cancer that may be similar to the hereditary type we have just discussed. The differentiating feature of this subtype, which appears before the menopause, is the occurrence in close relatives not only of early and bilateral breast cancer, but also of leukemia, brain tumors, sarcomas, and carcinomas of various organs, including lung, pancreas, and skin.

The exact mechanism underlying hereditary susceptibility to breast cancer is not known. Available evidence does suggest that some susceptible women may lack an enzyme (called estradiol hydroxylase) that would normally process the estrogen made by their own ovaries. With inadequate removal of estrogen, the slight excess remaining might serve to stimulate breast tissues to develop cancer.

Skin Cancer

While your genes may not predispose you specifically to skin cancer, they certainly do dictate the color of your skin and therefore your reaction to habitual exposure to sunlight. Furthermore, fair-skinned white people who sunburn easily develop cancers almost exclusively confined to the exposed parts (the face, head, neck, arms, and hands). Blacks remain remarkably resistant to the development of skin cancer, as do other races such as Orientals. Not surprisingly, the frequency of skin cancer differs markedly with geography. Fair-skinned individuals have a higher chance of dying of skin cancer if they live in one of the southern states in the United States. Cancer of the skin is also much more prevalent among outdoor workers such as farmers or sailors.

Some correlation exists between ethnic origin and the development of skin cancer. In people of Celtic ancestry, skin cancer may occur earlier and more frequently than would otherwise be expected. Hence, fair-skinned people of English, Welsh, or Irish descent would perhaps be more prone to it than others. Albinos, with a hereditary defect in skin and/or eye color, may have almost no pigment in their skin. After prolonged exposure to sunlight they invariably all develop cancer of the skin.

Cancer and Social Class

Cancer of the cervix occurs much more frequently among the poorer segment of the population and is associated with an earlier age of sexual intercourse, a larger number of sexual partners, poorer personal hygiene, poorer medical attention after childbirth, and infection with the herpes virus. It is of interest that the incidence of cancer of the cervix in white and black females of comparable socioeconomic status is very much the same.

Hereditary Disease and Cancer

A whole host of inherited disorders are associated with the subsequent development of cancer. Over 161 such examples are recognized, only a few of the most common being shown in the Table. It is not absolutely clear, even now, whether some of these hereditary conditions predispose to the development of cancer or whether they themselves and the growth of malignant tumors essentially reflect the same hereditary "fault." From the point of view of the individual with a hereditary disorder the matter is academic, since what is needed is the knowledge to *anticipate* malignant complications, to diagnose them early, and to effect permanent cures.

A number of well-known chromosomal disorders have a recognized association with subsequent development of var-

Do You Recognize Any of These Names?

If you or one of your parents have, or had, one of these or other hereditary tumors or conditions, you would be well advised to seek a consultation with a medical geneticist. (Organ commonly affected by cancer in parentheses.)

a. Tumors

Retinoblastoma (eye)

Neuroblastoma (adrenal gland)

Wilms' tumor (kidney — bilateral)

Acoustic neuroma (inner ear — bilateral)

Pheochromocytoma (involuntary nervous system, may be associated with thyroid cancer)

Teratoma (any organ)

Medulloblastoma (brain)

Basal cell carcinoma (skin)

Multiple endocrine adenomatosis (pancreas, thyroid, parathyroid, adrenal and other endocrine glands)

Keratoacanthoma (skin)

Melanoma (skin, eye)

b. Genetic Conditions

Familial polyposis of the colon (leads to cancer of the colon)

Peutz-Jegher's syndrome (associated with cancer of the colon and pigmentation of the mouth, lips, face, fingers, and toes)

Absent iris (eye) associated with kidney tumor (Wilms')

Gardner's syndrome (multiple tumors and intestinal polyps)

Albinism (skin)

Neurofibromatosis (nerves at any site)

Tuberous sclerosis (brain and other organs)

Xeroderma pigmentosum (skin)

Agammaglobulinemia (blood)

Ataxia telangiectasia (blood)

Bloom's syndrome (blood)

Fanconi's anemia (blood)

Alpha$_1$-antitrypsin deficiency (liver)

ious types of cancer. Take, for example, the most common chromosomal disorder, mongolism, where a ten- to twenty-fold increase in the frequency of acute leukemia is known to occur. When there is an extra #13 chromosome, called trisomy 13, or an extra X chromosome, called Klinefelter's syndrome, an increased incidence of leukemia has also been noted. Just as there is a higher frequency of sugar diabetes (diabetes mellitus) and thyroid disease in the parents of children with Down's syndrome, a higher frequency of various cancers in these same families has been observed.

In Klinefelter's syndrome (see Chapter 3), which causes males to develop feminine breasts after puberty, the frequency of cancer of the breast is about 66 times greater than in normal men; that is, a frequency similar to the incidence of cancer of the breast in women. In the condition associated with an extra chromosome #18 called trisomy 18, a higher frequency of kidney tumors (Wilms') has occurred. In a different kind of disorder where a piece of a chromosome is missing — and, in particular, a piece from the #13 chromosome — eye tumors or retinoblastoma has occurred. The suggestion has been that the gene controlling the cells that develop into the retinoblastoma might be on the piece of chromosome #13 that has been lost. Talking about deletions, one regularly associated deletion of a chromosome piece is that of #22. This abnormality is frequently associated with a chronic type of leukemia that mainly (though not only) affects adults. This abnormality apparently is found only in the blood-forming tissues and was observed in Philadelphia originally and is therefore called the Philadelphia chromosome.

There is a group of genetic conditions that are characterized by excessive breakage of chromosomes. Three well-known, though rare, disorders, called Bloom's syndrome, Fanconi's anemia, and Ataxia telangiectasia, are associated with as much as a 10 to 50 times increased risk of cancer. This group of genetic conditions are all inherited in a recessive manner (that is, both parents must be carriers), and there is a 25 percent chance that each child will be affected (see Chapter 5). It is interesting that an increased risk of leukemia has been noted not only in patients affected with, for example, Fanconi's anemia, but also in carriers of this disorder. One remarkable estimate is that among all persons dying with leukemia, one out of twenty is thought to be a carrier of Fanconi's anemia!

Some of these chromosomal-breakage syndromes have been associated with a disturbance of the immune system of the body, thus producing a greater susceptibility to infection. Indeed, there is a host of genetic disorders springing from a disturbed immune system, and here again the increased incidence of cancer is well established.

The Body's Defenders

Our bodies are defended, so to speak, by a variety of mechanisms including white blood cells, substances called antibodies, and a complex of other systems that all protect against invasion by "foreign" proteins, bacteria, viruses, and so on. The system that makes antibodies, which are protein molecules aimed at blocking the action of foreign proteins, has the ability to "recognize" an alien protein substance. The body, for example, recognizes its own cells by the specific protein coating each cell. Proteins in the blood stream, which are part of the immune system, may combine and inactivate foreign proteins. When a cancer appears, its cells have a different coat of protein from that of the other body cells, and our immune system is thought to recognize the appearance of this coating, thereby activating the mechanism to destroy the cancer cells. It has long been believed that failure of our immune system to destroy a developing cancer is the reason why the cancer continues to grow and eventually to spread and cause death. That is, the surveillance by the body defense mechanism becomes inadequate, as in old age. Of course, the specific types of protein that coat each cell in our body are genetically determined, as are those that circulate in the blood stream and are made in our lymph glands, spleen, and bone marrow.

Not unexpectedly then, when hereditary disorders of the immune system occur — and there are at least seven major such recognized immunodeficiency diseases — a higher frequency of cancer would be anticipated. This does indeed appear to be the case. Hence, if you or any of your relatives have been affected by this type of hereditary disease, the most careful and continual surveillance to detect cancer is advised.

Unfortunately, the problem has become even more complex. It turns out that patients who receive organ transplants, such as a kidney, require certain drugs to depress their immune systems so that the organ transplanted will not be rejected. Sadly, those individuals receiving organ transplants have a much greater frequency of malignancies of cells that make up the immune system. They do *not*, however, have a tendency toward developing any of the other common cancers. And this throws out of joint the theory highlighting the importance of surveillance by the immune system.

The most recent work has suggested that the body does indeed recognize the abnormal proteins coating the cancer cells and immediately makes antibodies aimed at destroying them, but the mechanism may go awry in that the antibodies act to protect the tumor instead of the person! Indeed, the notion has been advanced, again with supporting evidence, that these antibodies made to fight the cancer cells may even stimulate their growth! Where, where will it all end?

Changes in the Genes

A tumor can arise in any organ quite spontaneously and can be the first and last such tumor in a family. This is a nonhereditary form of cancer. Another situation is characterized by some mutation occurring in the genes resulting in the development of a specific tumor. While this tumor may not have occurred in the family before, its appearance signals a change in the genes that will now be transmitted from the affected person usually to half his or her children. Consideration of a few examples will serve to illustrate the point quite clearly.

In the specific eye cancer called retinoblastoma, if the tumor is found in both eyes, the victim may be saved by surgically removing the eyes plus the tumors. The children of such now blind individuals have a 50 percent chance of developing this same eye cancer. Strange and sad has been the more recent recognition that survivors of retinoblastoma in both eyes have an increased risk of developing bone cancer (osteosarcoma). When retinoblastoma occurs only in one eye, the chance that offspring of that individual will be affected is about 10 percent.

A similar story exists for Wilms' tumor of the kidney (and for other tumors, see the Table), where bilateral involvement of the kidneys is thought to be of the hereditary type. Of additional interest is the association of these tumors of the kidney with absence of the iris, the colored portion of the eye. It appears that the absent iris condition (called aniridia) may be associated in 33 percent of cases with the development of kidney tumors. Again, a similar situation exists for certain tumors of the adrenal gland (called neuroblastoma). A whole series of other rare cancers of a variety of different organ systems are known to affect siblings, first cousins, or be transmitted from one of the parents (see the Table). Simply discussing or enumerating tumor after tumor that has been noted in families could be confusing. Perhaps the best advice would be for you to consult a medical geneticist if any of the tumors listed in the Table have occurred in your close family. Since for almost every tumor there is a hereditary and a nonhereditary form, the geneticist may be helpful in either reassuring you or in providing you with certain tests, continued surveillance, and care.

Not infrequently, certain families are observed in which a whole variety of different types of tumors have occurred. For example, I recall one family whose various members had breast cancer, acute leukemia, brain tumors, cancers of the skin, pancreatic cancers, lung cancers, and even multiple tumors occurring in the same individual. If you are a member of such a family, then a consultation with a geneticist and an internist would be advantageous in setting up a system of careful surveillance through frequent medical checkups.

The fear of having cancer works to your disadvantage in making you act as though you don't really want to know. I cannot sufficiently emphasize how important it is for you to know your family history — to *know your genes*. Remember, most cancers, hereditary or nonhereditary, are curable if diagnosed early.

CHAPTER 20

Mental Illness and Heredity

MANY FIND MENTAL ILLNESS IN THE FAMILY much harder to deal with than physical problems. Perhaps this is in part due to fear, age-old stigmas and taboos, or to the frustration created by the invariably chronic nature of such an affliction. In recent years, however, treatment with drugs has made a significant difference.

There is a clear distinction between neuroses and the much more serious psychoses. The term *neurosis* implies some kind of deranged bodily function in the absence of an actual "physical" disease, which is dependent, in a way usually unknown to the afflicted person, on some kind of mental disturbance. Neurotic individuals — and we probably are all neurotic at least at some periods in our lives — may complain about an astounding variety of different symptoms that are all very real: aches and pains in various parts of the body, headaches, palpitations, breathlessness, loss of appetite, weakness, lethargy or fatigue, a feeling of pins and needles in the fingers, vomiting, diarrhea, constipation, excessive sweating, or a feeling of a lump in the throat. Mental disturbances may produce fear of heights, sounds, open or closed spaces, or there may be anxiety because of troublesome thoughts, inability to sleep sufficiently well, or compulsively repeated acts. There is no evidence that neuroses have a genetic basis. Through a shared environment, it could be anticipated that severely neurotic parents will be likely to have neurotic children.

This chapter will concentrate on the more severe types of mental illness classified as *psychoses*. Individuals who are psychotic have signs or symptoms that separate them from reality either constantly or intermittently. A number of different such disorders have been recognized, but the evidence for a genetic basis is important only in two: schizophrenia and manic depression.

Schizophrenia

The term *schizophrenia* was first introduced about 60 years ago to describe a splitting between thought and emotional responses — giving rise to the idea of "split personality." Today, schizophrenia is considered to be a disorder of thought processes and expresses itself as a disorder of feeling, through inappropriate behavior and an increasing withdrawal from interpersonal contacts. There are various typical symptoms. A person may believe he is God, dispensing blessings, charity, or even punishment. Patients may be hallucinated, walking around intently listening to voices they maintain they are hearing. These voices, they say, are giving them instructions to perform certain acts that may even be murder. Some may become totally withdrawn, hardly moving a limb. They may stand with an arm in the air or in some other unusual posture for hours at a time — a so-called catatonic state. Other patients may become paranoid, insisting that someone or many people are out to kill them or to persecute them, and so on.

Schizophrenia is common and is thought to occur in about 1 in every 100 individuals in the United States. The first episode may occur sometime between adolescence and fifty years of age, most patients being diagnosed in their twenties. Both males and females are equally affected, although there appear to be more males among the young who suffer from it.

Is Schizophrenia an Inherited Disorder?

If schizophrenia is indeed as common as 1 in every 100 individuals, then in the United States alone there is a staggering figure of over 2 million affected persons! The likelihood is that while this figure may be true, many of the persons are affected only periodically, with mild symptoms, and easily treated. Those who are severely affected come to the attention of psychiatrists or society fairly quickly.

You will not be surprised, then, at how often people come for genetic counseling concerned because of schizophrenia in their family, wondering whether either they or their offspring may ultimately develop it. There have been simply endless studies to determine whether schizophrenia is hereditary or not. Three groups of studies have provided the best data: families of schizophrenics, twin studies, and adopted children.

Schizophrenia in the Family

Reliable data on familial schizophrenia took a long time to formulate since definitions of schizophrenia have varied appreciably, especially from country to country. Nevertheless information available today clearly indicates that there is an increased likelihood of schizophrenia occurring when someone in the family is affected. The estimates of such occurrences are summarized in the Table. Parents of schizophrenics are affected themselves about 5 percent of the time. A brother or sister of a schizophrenic has an average risk of about 8.7 percent for developing schizophrenia, and so on through the Table.

Schizophrenia in Twins

Enormous efforts have been made to study twins with all kinds of genetic disease (see Chapter 26). The idea of course is that if the disorder is genetic then there would be a high likelihood that identical twins would have or would develop the same disorder. The data on identical twins have shown that both twins have been affected in about 47 percent of cases, although there has been marked variation in reported studies (15 to 85 percent). The 47 percent figure for schizophrenia affecting both identical twins is strikingly higher than the 2 to 10 percent occurrence rate noted for nonidentical twins. Many critics have maintained that identical twins reared in the same home may be subject to the same kinds of pressures and environmental variables and have therefore questioned the significance of those studies.

Frequency of Schizophrenia Among the Relatives of Schizophrenics

Relationship to Schizophrenic	Chance of Having Schizophrenia (Estimates in %)
Parent	5.1
Brother or sister	8.7
Identical twin	47.0
Child (one parent schizophrenic)	12.0
Child (both parents schizophrenic)	39.0
Uncle or aunt	2.0
Nephew or niece	2.2
First cousin	2.9
Unrelated (general population)	0.9

Schizophrenia in Adopted Children

Since the family environment could potentially affect the upbringing of identical twins, thereby possibly influencing the development of schizophrenia, researchers led by Professor Seymour Kety at the Massachusetts General Hospital devised elaborate studies to examine adopted children to determine the frequency of schizophrenia in children removed early in life from their home and family. These adoption studies were done in Denmark by American and Danish psychiatrists in collaboration. Denmark was selected because the records of adoptions and of episodes of schizophrenia and other vital records are so magnificently collected and kept.

The goal of the first study was to determine the frequency of schizophrenia in the adopted children of parents, one or both of whom were schizophrenic. These figures were compared to the frequency of schizophrenia in the natural offspring of the families of adopting parents. The researchers found that schizophrenia among the adopted offspring of schizophrenics was three times that found in the natural offspring of adopting parents. Later studies concluded by demonstrating the same frequency of schizophrenia in children of schizophrenic parents who were themselves adopted early in life, compared to those who were raised by schizophrenic parents themselves. Moreover, schizophrenia was found to occur among the adopted offspring of normal parents (without schizophrenia) at about the same rate as noted in the general population.

To exclude the effects of the environment in the womb or influences surrounding birth or early mothering, another study was devised to determine the frequency of schizophrenia in adopted offspring who had the same fathers but different mothers. This study concluded by showing that significantly more offspring of the same father with schizophrenia had the disorder than did matched control groups.

The adoption studies were meant to separate out the hereditary from the environmental effects on child rearing. One unexpected observation was the slightly higher level of mental illness in those parents who adopted children who later became schizophrenic, as compared to parents adopting children who did not become schizophrenic. The significance of this finding remains unclear at present.

Confounding Factors

The inexorable conclusion from these remarkable, painstaking family studies is that genetic influences are involved in schizophrenia. It is equally obvious that schizophrenia, like mental retardation, represents a variety of different disorders and causes, and consequently different patterns of inheritance can be expected. As for environmental influences, some evidence suggests that childhood schizophrenia develops more often in those children who have had complications during and immediately after the birth process than in their brothers or sisters who had normal births. Moreover, the offspring of parents of whom at least one is a schizophrenic have been noted to have a higher frequency of fetal death or death in the newborn period. A curious observation was made by some researchers who noted that when the sex of children born to women in hospital for schizophrenia was examined, there were no males if symptoms of the schizophrenia in the mother had occurred within one month of conception of that infant. They further noted that if the schizophrenic episode began within two or three months before or even after conception, there were significantly fewer males among the babies born as well as an increased frequency of stillbirths, malformations, and even birth defects! Some studies draw attention to the point that schizophrenics themselves are more likely to have been born during the winter months, from January to March.

It has long been noted that certain drugs that cause hallucinations, such as LSD, may precipitate schizophrenia — perhaps in the predisposed individual. Some psychiatrists have separated out their psychotic patients into those in whom no cause whatsoever can be suggested or found — called nonorganic — and those where some suggestion or sign of abnormality in brain function, such as mild mental retardation, limited speech, and so on, can be determined — called organic. Evidence has shown that children or adolescents with deviant behavior gross enough to be called psychotic probably include a number with dysfunction of the brain. This insight shed some light on a remarkable observation made some years ago. Dr. William Pollin noticed that if only one twin of an identical twin pair was psychotic, he or she was lighter in birth weight and was more likely to have been exposed to damage interfering with brain development. He also found that many of the affected psychotic twins had some suggestion of brain dysfunction.

Susceptibility to Schizophrenia?

There have been a number of studies aimed at determining the susceptibility of individuals to the development of schizophrenia. Using the computer to analyze patients' speech patterns, it has been observed that schizophrenics have a sense of disorientation and chaotic thought in association with apparent certain defenses against confusion and discomfort. These speech pattern analyses are being applied to relatives of schizophrenics who are not overtly affected.

Another approach has been the analysis of eye movements, as the eyes track a moving pendulum. The study concentrated on scoring how smoothly the eyes move in response to the pendulum, the number of times they stopped when they should have been following its movement, or the number of times the eyes moved ahead of it. Deviations occurred more frequently among schizophrenics than normal individuals. Of particular interest was the observation that "abnormal" eye movements in tracking the pendulum were noted in many more asymptomatic relatives of schizophrenics than in persons with no schizophrenia in the family.

Manic Depressive Illness

Depression is a very common symptom that affects each of us at some time in our lives. Depression may, for example, occur perfectly normally after sad events such as the death of a loved one, personal illness, or family problems and is not usually considered a neurosis. When it occurs without any relationship to obvious problems, then it may well be part of anxiety neurosis. We will not discuss depression of this sort but rather concentrate on the very much more serious disorder of manic depression: a psychosis associated with extreme elation or profound depression, either of which dominates the patient's entire mental life in cycles.

Individuals with manic depression may have alternating episodes of mania or extreme uncontrollable excitement and deep despair. Some patients have only episodes of mania; others only depression. Each form has special characteristics.

The patients with the manic phase of the disorder are characterized by an extremely elated though unstable mood, flights of ideas, and tremendous physical and mental activity. I have never forgotten a particular patient with mania that I saw 20 years ago while still a medical student. She had been a perfectly healthy young woman with a normal, happy disposition. One day out of the blue she suddenly developed manic excitement, became extremely restless, talking and screaming continuously, her elation reaching points of ecstasy at times. She expressed peculiar ideas declaring that she was acting under orders of God, with whom she had spoken. At the time she was admitted, she insisted that the doctor kiss her and berated him when he refused. She could hardly finish a sentence, moving from a description of what God instructed her to do, to active efforts to embrace doctors in attendance, exposing her body and inviting anyone walking by to make love to her, and became extremely excited and angry when such efforts failed. She then smashed crockery, tore her bed clothes, broke glass, and flung things at other patients. She ultimately recovered completely, but had amnesia for the particular period during which she was ill.

The profoundly depressed individuals have difficulty in thinking and may have associated depressed physical activity. They may be suicidal, have hallucinations, hear voices, feel they are being persecuted, and hardly talk at all. They may be careless in their dress and, in extreme cases, even soil their clothes with urine or feces.

Is Manic Depressive Illness Inherited?

Close to 1 in 100 in the general population have or will develop manic depressive illness. A larger amount of the general population than one would suppose have or will develop manic depressive symptoms. There is a clear indication that it runs in families, with females outnumbering males. As in schizophrenia, identical twins are more often prone to manic depression than nonidentical twins. The symptoms within a given family are usually similar.

The pattern of transmission, however, is not entirely clear. There are probably more types of manic depression than the two main forms we mentioned: bipolar, in which manic episodes are interspersed with depression; and unipolar, with unremitting depression. It is very significant that families with incidences of bipolar manic depression have shown an inheritance pattern typical of a sex-linked dominant disorder (see Chapter 5), which simply means that many more females than males are affected and that father to son transmission of this disorder does not occur in these particular families. A female child of a parent with the bipolar type of manic depression might theoretically at least have as much as a 50 percent risk of developing it. The available data only *suggest* that for the unipolar type the mode of inheritance is dominant, so that the 50 percent risk is still problematical. Much work has still to be done, though it is clear that in one certain type of manic depressive disease heredity plays its eternal role.

Infantile Autism

Professionals are still debating the origins of this serious disorder. Many have considered it a form of schizophrenia that simply becomes evident during the first year or so of life. Others point to the withdrawal and other symptoms of children with certain forms of mental retardation and seek to put autism in one of these categories. Others even deny any correlation between infantile autism and mental retardation. Notwithstanding problems of definition, the characteristic, and devastating, signs are only too well known.

Most cases are probably evident at birth, but the hints are so subtle they are frequently missed. Both parents and doctor may fail to notice the lack of eye-to-eye contact with the mother when feeding, or the lack of anticipation of and responsiveness to being picked up. Other typical signs include: extreme self-isolation; aloofness; withdrawal; apparent insensitivity to pain; treating people as objects (the child may stand on the head of a playmate); failure to develop language; repetitive body movement, rocking or hand-flapping; self-mutilation; head banging, and so on.

The best evidence points to the cause being a complex dysfunction in the brain stem that interferes with the perception and reception of every kind of sensation or stimulus, from pain to speech.

While a few researchers have postulated a genetic basis for infantile autism, there are really no convincing supporting data.

CHAPTER 21

Diabetes

EVERY ADULT IN OUR WESTERN CIVILIZATION and elsewhere has probably heard of diabetes mellitus or sugar diabetes. And small wonder, since according to recent estimates there are some 200 million diabetics in the world.

Most people know that diabetics have a high level of glucose, or sugar, in the blood that spills over into the urine, and that they have a relative or absolute lack of insulin, the hormone secreted by the pancreas. The insulin deficiency creates two major problems. The first is a biochemical disturbance in body chemistry creating a high blood glucose level that changes the body's fat and protein chemistry. These changes may lead to diabetic coma and death if untreated. The second major danger approaches slowly over many years in the large and small blood vessels of the diabetic. Atherosclerosis (see Chapter 18) may be accelerated and disease of small blood vessels, particularly affecting the eyes and kidneys, brings on blindness, kidney failure, and possibly death. The longer the duration of certain types of diabetes, the more likely are these blood vessel changes to occur. By and large, as a group, diabetics at present face a diminished life expectancy and daily confront the possibility of disaster. On the other hand, you may know individuals with diabetes who have been well for many, many decades.

History

Diabetes has been recognized for a few thousand years. While it is not known exactly who first described diabetes, we know that it existed some 3000 years ago in Egypt. Early Chinese medical writings also described a condition that was almost certainly diabetes. Physicians in India around 400 B.C.E. observed the sweetness of the urine as well as the association between obesity and diabetes and the familial nature of the disorder. The disease was named about the beginning of the Christian era by the Romans Aretaeus and Celsus, who called it diabetes (siphon) and mellitus or melli (honey or sweet). This was about 70 C.E. That the sweetness in the urine was due to sugar was only recognized late in the eighteenth century. In 1859, the great French physiologist Claude Bernard demonstrated the increased glucose content of blood in the diabetic patient. About ten years later, the areas of the pancreas that we know today secrete insulin were noted to be abnormal. This led in 1889 to experiments that first produced diabetes in dogs by removing the pancreas.

These latter observations gave tremendous impetus to efforts made to prepare extracts from the pancreas, which were then used to attempt to correct the deficiency in the disease. Continuous success using extracts prepared from dog pancreas to reduce the blood glucose level was achieved in 1921 in Toronto by Canadian workers. Long-acting insulin was introduced about 1936. Extracts of pancreas of course contain insulin. The chemical structure of human insulin was only established in 1960. In 1967, in Chicago, a large molecule (called proinsulin) was detected in the blood from which insulin is derived. Not unexpectedly, proinsulin, too, is under genetic control.

When Is Diabetes, Diabetes?

It is a simple matter to diagnose overt diabetes in an individual complaining of typical symptoms and having sugar in the urine plus an elevated blood sugar. There are various states of diabetes, and it is not at all inevitable for one state to progress to another. The first state is overt diabetes, as mentioned. Second, an individual who has no symptoms of diabetes may be found to have elevated blood glucose levels only after a meal or after a glucose-tolerance test. (This test involves giving a person a "load" of sugar either by mouth or intravenously, and measuring how high the blood sugar level goes over a three- to five-hour period.) This second state is called asymptomatic or chemical diabetes. The third state, called latent or stress diabetes, occurs in a person who has a normal glucose-tolerance test, but who was diabetic at some time in the past during a period of stress, for example, during pregnancy, during serious infection, when very much overweight, or in association with a heart attack or serious burns. The fourth state is one of truly potential diabetes, signaled by a medical history of a female who has given birth to a baby weighing more than ten pounds. This state cannot easily be diagnosed with certainty, nor can accurate predictions be made that such a woman would necessarily become diabetic.

How Large a Problem?

About 4 in every 100 people in the United States have diabetes. Only about 2 in every 100, however, have been diagnosed — that is, approximately 4 million persons in the United States. The other 2 in every 100, approximately 4 million more, have diabetes with few or no symptoms, and which can only be diagnosed by glucose-tolerance tests.

While diabetes occurs in all countries, its frequency varies considerably, undoubtedly reflecting environmental, cultural, and, probably, genetic differences. It is rare in the Eskimo, is incredibly common among certain American Indians, such as the Pima in Arizona, where up to 50 percent of the population may develop the disease. The incidence of diabetes in the Pima Indians is rivaled by that of Asian Indians who emigrated to South Africa, or in Orientals, especially the Japanese, and these cases differ appreciably from the diabetes seen in the United States, the United Kingdom, and Europe.

The frequency of diabetes is increasing for a number of reasons. The population is growing and people are living longer. (About four of every five diabetics are over forty-five years of age.) Carefully treated diabetics are living longer and, as a consequence, have children, something they may not have been able to do so often many years ago. All of these children will inherit the gene for or susceptibility to diabetes. Finally, obesity, which appears to precipitate or aggravate the disease, is also increasing, thereby making more potential diabetics clinically obvious. Among the diabetics, 85 percent are, or were at one time, overweight.

Who Should Be Tested?

Since it is not feasible to do complete blood tests on virtually all adults in the population, it is worthwhile focusing on individuals who are likely to have a higher risk of diabetes. Blood glucose tests should be done at least yearly on the relatives of diabetics, who have a higher risk, on overweight individuals at every annual checkup, especially if they are over forty, and on mothers who have had babies with high birthweight (over ten pounds). Such women clearly have a higher risk of developing diabetes. Everyone having an operation, a preemployment physical, or an annual checkup should have a routine test for diabetes even if they have no known family history of it.

The Causes of Diabetes

One becomes a diabetic for both hereditary and environmental reasons — usually a combination of both. Obviously, destruction of the pancreas because of cancer, serious infection, inflammation, or disease would be a cause. Certain diseases of other hormone-producing glands, such as the pituitary, may be correlated with the onset of diabetes. It may be precipitated, on occasion, by the intake of drugs, including cortisone, some diuretics (pills to rid the body of water), and, possibly, by some of the sex-hormone combination pills.

Genetics or Environment

The assumptions were, and still are, that some people have a genetic susceptibility to diabetes that becomes stimulated by their life-styles and their environment.

Obesity

The prevalence of obesity in certain populations increases the incidence of diabetes. It is well established that glucose intolerance increases with body weight. One study on this correlation involved the brothers and sisters of diabetics who developed the disease mainly between their third and fifth decades. The siblings who were not obese were five times less likely to become diabetic than those who were obese. (On the other hand, among the South African Bantus, the most obese women have the *lowest* rate of diabetes.)

It is still not clear whether obesity itself or something in the diet is the most important factor. The best evidence implicates the fats in our diet. Evidence that high sugar intake is equally guilty has not been generally accepted. Suggestions about the importance of chromium deficiency in the diet and lack of vegetable fiber require further evaluation. Meanwhile, it appears that the influence of obesity on diabetes is greater in those presumed to carry a genetic susceptibility to this disease. It is interesting that the incidence of diabetes fell off considerably in Japan during World War II and the years of food privation that followed.

Studies of immigrant populations have given interesting results along these lines. One of the best was done in Israel where the frequency of diabetes in Yemenite Jews who had recently arrived was compared to that of Jews who had lived in Israel for 25 years or more. The latter were found to have approximately 40 times as many diabetics among them as the newest immigrants. The Indians of South Africa are another example. They are reported to have a frequency of diabetes some ten times higher than that found in the Punjab where their ancestors hailed from. Similarly, a four- to twentyfold increase in diabetes was noted for Polynesian peoples in the Pacific, compared to those living on the New Zealand mainland.

Reflecting either dietary influences or genetic susceptibilities, high blood fat levels (cholesterol and triglycerides) or high uric acid levels (causing gout) are known to be associated with diabetes.

Sex, Age, and the Number of Children

For reasons that are not entirely certain, involvement of males or females has varied over the years. For example, an excess of males was replaced by an excess of females diagnosed as diabetic at the beginning of the twentieth century. These past 20 years, however, direction of change has moved back to an excess of men. Possibly, changing fashions in family size and variations in the frequency of obesity contribute to changes in sex ratios.

We have already noted that the incidence of overt, as well as clinical, diabetes increases with advancing age. Indeed, the criteria for the diagnosis of diabetes suggest that by the age of one hundred, over 90 percent of individuals would have at least chemical diabetes.

In some societies, there are indications that the more children a woman has, the more likely is she to develop diabetes. The implication is that pregnancy itself is a diabetes-causing factor. Whether there is a genetic component to this tendency remains unclear.

Infection

The idea that diabetes could result from an infection might surprise you. It is, however, well known that in animals diabetes can be induced by viruses such as the Coxsackie B4 virus or the foot-and-mouth virus. It is hard to prove that diabetes in a human has been induced by a virus. It can always be argued that the virus acted as a stress phenomenon precipitating diabetes in someone so predisposed. However, there are some data that show a seasonal variation in the incidence of new cases of insulin-dependent diabetes in individuals under thirty years of age, the peaks coming in September and December, suggesting strongly the machination of a virus. Coxsackie B4 virus has definitely been implicated in these seasonal peaks. High levels of antibodies against that particular virus have been unexpectedly prevalent in juvenile diabetes patients. Children damaged in the womb by German measles have a higher risk of developing diabetes later in life.

In diabetes with an onset in childhood, antibodies to the child's own pancreas have been repeatedly detected in the blood. It is not known whether infection of the pancreas initiated the process; but it is known that in certain diseases, the body responds by making antibodies to its own organs, such as the thyroid or adrenal glands, and such conditions are frequently associated with diabetes.

Simultaneous development of the disease in brothers and sisters is another clue suggesting an infectious agent. There is one family I know of that suffered three children developing diabetes within three months of each other. In spite of such evidence, however, the matter becomes increasingly complicated when you recognize that some of us may be genetically predisposed to certain infections and, in that way, have a higher risk of developing diabetes. At this point, it might be useful to consider the known genetic aspects.

Genetic Factors

Blood Groups We discussed elsewhere (Chapter 6) diseases associated with specific blood groups or tissue types. Most recently, evidence has been presented that individuals with groups HLA-B8 or BW15 have about 2.5 times more chance of developing so-called juvenile insulin-dependent diabetes, early in life, than young people with other blood groups. The best available data suggest that the sibling of this type of juvenile diabetic has a 10 to 11 percent chance of developing diabetes if he or she has either the HLA-B8 or BW15 blood group; if both blood groups are present, then the risk is about 20 percent. The two blood groups under discussion occur with significant frequency only in patients with juvenile-onset diabetes. This kind of diabetes is especially characterized by an early age of onset, a normal body weight, the presence of antibodies to the individual's own pancreas, and other specific features of the pancreas seen under the microscope.

An association between the juvenile type of insulin-dependent diabetes and other HLA types DW3 and DW4, which is stronger than that described above, has very recently been recognized. About 80 percent of juvenile diabetics have been noted to have these blood or tissue types. How all these blood groups make a person susceptible to insulin-dependent diabetes is still totally unknown. It is interesting to note in one study that over 70 percent of children with birth defects due to German measles and who developed diabetes had HLA-B8 types. Finally, even the seasonal peaks of diabetes are now being explained by evidence showing that juvenile diabetics usually have HLA-B8 blood or tissue types. The current view is that individuals who develop juvenile-onset diabetes have genes associated with the HLA-B8 type, which make them susceptible to certain viruses. The cells of the pancreas that make insulin (B-cells) may be more susceptible to these viruses, which cause their destruction directly or through the antibodies made by the body to "fight" against them.

In the past, both members of a pair of identical twins were noted to develop diabetes in about 50 percent of cases, in contrast to about 9 percent for nonidentical twins. Most recently, it has been noted that the age at which such studies in diabetes are done is particularly relevant. The figures on average suggest concordance (both affected) for identical twins in 71 percent of cases. If, however, identical twins aged fifty and over were studied, both twins were found to be diabetic in 100 percent of cases.

The latest data suggest that once one identical twin has diabetes, in the vast majority of cases, the second twin will develop it within three years. In a few cases, it may take as long as ten years for the second twin to become diabetic. The present evidence indicates that the chances are extremely small for a co-twin also to develop diabetes more than ten years after the other twin.

As might be expected, a family history of diabetes is found much more often in cases where both twins have it (45 percent) than when only one twin has the disease (17 percent), implying that the concordant twins have a strong genetic component to their illness. A moment's reflection, however, will lead you to conclude that a positive family history of diabetes will increase as the family, in general, and the diabetic, in particular, gets older. Unexpectedly, perhaps, identical twin studies clearly suggest that genetic factors cannot entirely explain the diabetes of the juvenile-onset insulin-dependent type, but may be the explanation for this disorder in older individuals.

In general, there are two kinds of diabetes — one requiring insulin and the other being managed with diet or pills (oral hypoglycemic drugs). Individuals with juvenile-onset (less than forty years of age) diabetes most often, but not always, require insulin for treatment, whereas diabetes diagnosed after forty years of age can frequently be managed without it.

When One Parent Is Diabetic

Very recently, it has become clear that the rarer juvenile-onset diabetics who do not have to depend on insulin are similar to individuals with the same kind of diabetes diagnosed after forty years of age. It is this type of the disease that has now been recognized as having genetic origins. The best available data document this most important conclusion. By and large, when one parent has this type of diabetes, the risk appears to be 50 percent for each child. You will recognize, then, that it is a dominant form of inheritance (see Chapter 5).

It is known that diabetics of this type may have remarkably few complications even after decades of illness. The implication is that it is basically a very different type of diabetes from the juvenile-onset insulin-dependent disease, which is characterized by the severest of complications. The risk for an individual developing diabetes when one parent has diabetes that began in childhood and has required insulin continuously is much less, about 11 percent.

When Both Parents Are Diabetic

It is obvious that the risk of developing diabetes when both parents have it will depend upon the type of diabetes each parent has. There are no useful data to form the basis of a reliable opinion when both parents have juvenile-onset insulin-dependent diabetes. There are also not a great deal of data concerning the offspring of two diabetic parents who have early onset but are not insulin-dependent. What information is available suggests that in about two-thirds of such marriages, diabetic offspring resulted. An exact reliable risk figure for each pregnancy for such a couple cannot yet be given. The matter is not yet closed.

Diabetes Associated with Other Genetic Disorders

Diabetes occurs with significantly increased frequency in individuals with certain chromosomal abnormalities such as Down's syndrome, Klinefelter's syndrome, and Turner's syndrome (see Chapters 2 and 3). While the exact explanation for these observations is not known, one intriguing possibility is that affected individuals and their parents have a genetic predisposition to develop antibodies to one or more of their own organs (e.g., thyroid). Antibodies so produced might damage the cells in the pancreas that produce insulin, thereby inducing the diabetic state.

An endless list of other genetic disorders or syndromes exists where diabetes or intolerance to glucose is known. Cystic fibrosis, Huntington's chorea, and certain types of muscular dystrophy are but three representatives of this long list. The mechanism for the development of diabetes is likely to be somewhat different in each.

Conclusion

Advice about the risks of inheriting diabetes based on data available years ago is now probably incorrect. To give reliable advice, it is necessary to analyze carefully the family history, to investigate the tissues and blood types, to ascertain the degree of glucose intolerance and, perhaps, make some other tests. The sort of complications that seem to be in store for a diabetic probably reflect the genetic type of his or her disease. We know, at least, that for one type of diabetic many decades of life without complications are often possible.

We have established as causes direct hereditary transmission, interaction between genes and environment, as well as purely acquired ones such as surgical removal of the pancreas or some fateful infection.

Diabetes may be mild or severe, require insulin or not, have few or many attendant complications. We know also that inherited susceptibility to infection, obesity, or heart disease can tip the scales. Clearly, much has yet to be learned about this ailment.

CHAPTER 22

Treating Genetic Disease

How, you may ask, can one treat a hereditary disease? Is it not irrevocable and irreversible? Can such a disorder be remedied in any fashion?

True, it is not yet possible to *cure* a genetic disorder, though some progress has been made toward that end. What *is* eminently feasible is the *treatment* of such disabilities. Research has made leaps and bounds in this area of medicine. People can be helped tremendously; their lives can be saved by recognition of hazardous situations. Many people in this category live entirely normal lifespans. The goal of treatment is either to prevent a genetic disorder from becoming manifest or to minimize its adverse effects.

What are the treatments possible for an array of hereditary disorders?

Diet

The relation of certain foods to aggravation of hereditary disorders is no longer in question. As one example, very many blacks are born lacking a certain intestinal enzyme, called lactase, necessary for the digestion of milk and milk products. This may not become obvious until late childhood or even until adulthood. These individuals suffer diarrhea after drinking milk or eating milk products. They can lead normal lives if they avoid these products.

For certain genetic disorders, some foods prove toxic or even lethal. Both mental retardation and death may be the result. Professor Y. E. Hsia of Yale has listed dietary measures for various diseases, describing the therapy in categories. Using his perspective, we shall take them up one by one.

Augmentation

Certain foods and liquids can be used to protect a patient against biochemical disorders. Some of the instructions are remarkably easy to follow. In sickle cell anemia the blood cells become sickle-shaped when dehydration occurs. It is therefore very important for the patient to drink a fair amount of water. Water is also essential in the treatment of cystinuria, the genetic condition that produces kidney stones. The taking of alkalis provides additional help in preventing stone formation in both kidney and bladder. A number of hereditary disorders involve low blood sugar, or hypoglycemia, and simply having sweet foods around may protect one against the complications of the disease.

Some biochemical disorders require much more than simple dietary therapy. Some sugars, such as glucose and galactose, can cause serious problems for persons with hereditary disorders of carbohydrate metabolism. For a baby with such a condition (galactosemia), the milk sugar galactose may cause brain damage, cirrhosis of the liver, cataracts, and even death soon after birth. All these are preventable by strict dietary exclusion from the very first days of life, and even better, by excluding these sugars from the diet of the prospective mother. Prenatal diagnosis is very important here, since treatment of the fetus via the mother is possible.

In a condition called fructose intolerance the body is unable to tolerate sugars in fruit, therapy is facilitated because the patient often develops an aversion to sweet-tasting foods.

Cutting out foods containing cholesterol, such as eggs and saturated fats, is an important maneuver in treating some hereditary heart and blood disorders, as we have mentioned earlier. There is even a disorder involving a chemical related to chlorophyll that may cause serious nerve damage and blindness. The removal of all green fruits and vegetables from the diet may prevent or at least ameliorate the disease.

Restriction and Substitution

There is a real problem when an essential food is toxic to a patient with a hereditary disease. Deprivation of that essential food can lead to serious malnutrition, failure to grow, and even death. Substitution of synthetic products may become essential. The condition called PKU (phenylketonuria) is the best example here. As we have said, the blood and urine of newborn infants is routinely tested for PKU, and diagnosis during the first days of life, plus immediate initiation of a restricted diet, will easily allow such children to develop normally and without the severe mental retardation, eczema, seizures and other complications of PKU.

What has to be restricted is a certain essential amino acid called phenylalanine that is present in all high-grade proteins and is necessary to the body in the making of all its proteins. By careful regulation of this amino acid, plus frequent monitoring and substitution of synthetic protein, it is possible to treat the affected child successfully. It does take, however, the most sophisticated care in a major medical center. Fortunately, the severity of the diet restriction can be eased up at about the time the child starts going to school. But many parents will attest to the enormous strain and emotional drain this therapy puts on the family. The unnatural diet deprives the child of many foods he or she wants to eat; and some of the synthetic substitutes have a definitely unpleasant taste. The continuous attention by the doctor, the repetitive taking of blood samples, the special caution that must surround the child, all take their toll. But there is no doubt that without such careful dietary treatment, almost all PKU children will develop severe brain damage and be untrainable as well as uneducable.

Once the patient with PKU grows up, marries, and decides to have children, an additional dimension of care is needed. In the past, such eventualities were rare indeed. Nowadays, if the diet has been properly controlled, they will probably marry and bear offspring. In past experiences, virtually 100 percent of their children were mentally retarded. Now it is recognized that by keeping a PKU woman on a restricted diet when pregnant, one can ensure that the toxic phenylalanine in her blood stream will not damage the brain of the fetus. It does appear clear that once brain damage has become evident in PKU, it is irreversible.

Wilson's disease, which is due to a defect in copper metabolism resulting in a tremendous overstorage of copper in the brain and liver, is another example of a disorder that can be treated with dietary restrictions. All foods with high copper content such as cherries, chocolate, or beef must be cut out completely. Drugs to rid the body of copper must be taken as well.

Supplementation and Replacement

Specific dietary supplements may be lifesaving in the treatment of hereditary disease. There is a host of chemical disorders in which amino acids or protein supplementation is crucial. Another type of supplementation in the treatment of diabetes insipidus involves water plus a hormone. Diabetes insipidus, a sex-linked disorder carried by females but affecting only males, renders the kidney unable to concentrate urine. (A different sort of diabetes from sugar diabetes.) The patient passes excessive quantities of urine, becomes dehydrated, and, eventually, may die. Water supplementation temporarily saves the day. But a replacement is also needed: the kidney's inability to deal with the urine is due to deficiency of a hormone made in the pituitary gland at the base of the brain. Medical research has made it possible to obtain this hormone in powder form; the patient is given it to use as snuff. From the nose the powder is absorbed into the blood stream and circulates to the kidney where it enables that organ to concentrate the urine.

Vitamins added to the diet may be extremely important in heredity disorders of the metabolism. In diseases such as cystic fibrosis, for example, in which the fat is not properly absorbed, the fat-soluble vitamins A, D, E, and K will also not be absorbed. Deficiency of vitamin K shows itself in excessive bleeding and bruising. In some complex biochemical disabilities, vitamin supplementation will stimulate compensatory chemical reactions in the body and overcome the basic derangement. Since vitamins are vital to certain body reactions, sometimes massive doses are needed.

Success was achieved in the treatment of a fetus having a biochemical disorder, called methylmalonic aciduria, by administration of enormous amounts of vitamin B_{12} directly to the mother (see Chapter 16). This is the ideal we all seek: to avert the need for abortion by safe treatment of the fetus still in the womb. It is with this goal in mind that much work needs to be done to avoid the trauma of abortion and to ensure that wanted children are born normal and healthy.

In the case of cystic fibrosis, the most common genetic killer of children in the white population, much more than vitamin supplementation is needed. While it is mainly characterized by recurrent lung infection, it is also associated with deficient secretion by the pancreas of enzymes necessary for digestion. An extract of the actual enzymes is usually administered by mouth to cystic fibrosis patients — they may take as many as ten tablets with each meal for life. This does not cure the disease, but usually enables the patient to have close to a normal bowel habit.

Treatment with Drugs

A few examples will serve to illustrate the kinds of drugs used to mitigate some genetic diseases. A very large number are used.

The thyroid gland may be extremely underactive at birth, the causes, on occasion, being hereditary. Simply initiating treatment with thyroid hormone will prevent the child from becoming mentally retarded. This treatment must be lifelong. In another hereditary disorder, the adrenal gland fails to manufacture cortisone: a situation that could cause death in early infancy. Again, the situation is remedied by administering cortisone for life. Certain forms of gout are hereditary, and the use of specific drugs will block the formation of uric acid, thereby preventing the excruciating attacks of pain. In Wilson's disease, mentioned earlier, a drug related to penicillin, called penicillamine, is used to flush the excess copper out through the urine. In hereditary conditions with high blood cholesterol, nicotinic acid or a drug called Atromid-S (clofibrate) can be used to lower blood cholesterol by interfering with its production.

Even in disorders in which there may be an extra chromosome or one too few, the affected person may be appreciably helped by drug treatment (see Chapters 2 and 3).

Modifying the Internal Environment

This is an approach that again fails to cure any genetic disorder but, by modifying the body chemistry, may save life or tremendously improve its quality. Very recently, a remarkably effective new treatment was discovered for a rare but usually fatal disease affecting mainly the skin and the bowel, called by the long name acrodermatitis enteropathica. Before 1972, children with this disorder (inherited from both parents equally) frequently died. The discovery was made in England by Dr. E. J. Moynahan that zinc taken by mouth remedies the problem in the bowel and the skin as long as the patient continues to take the medication. Hence, a previously fatal genetic disease, while not cured, can be managed in such a way as to ensure a probable normal life expectancy, and this without even knowing the basic defect involved.

Some of the hereditary disorders afflicting newborns may be so severe as to cause immediate coma and death if not recognized in time. In this group, biochemical products have accumulated in the fetus that are toxic and rapidly kill the infant. Treatment, which may be astonishingly effective, consists of changing or modifying the internal environment of the baby immediately, for example, by literally exchanging the whole blood volume and replacing it with blood from a donor. The toxic product can also be removed from the infant's body by a variety of techniques, including kidney dialysis.

Treatment by a Replacement

The blood-clotting factor missing in hemophilia (Factor VIII), which causes the victims to go on bleeding after receiving even a small cut, a tooth extraction, or merely a bump or laceration, can be obtained and concentrated from donated blood plasma and put into blood products called cryoprecipitates. While they do not cure hemophilia, they make a tremendous difference to patients with it. The trouble is that it costs about $12,000 a year to obtain sufficient cryoprecipitates for treatment per patient. In addition to the cost, their production takes enormous quantities of blood, and human blood is extremely scarce and needed in a large number of surgical and medical situations. Funding for research is urgently needed to enable the missing blood factor to be made synthetically.

Replacement of proteins is important in the treatment of many genetic disorders. In one rare condition, again confined like hemophilia to males, the child may not be able to make the chemical called gamma globulin, which protects the body against infection. It therefore has to be administered for life.

A missing enzyme causes a large number of hereditary handicaps. The problem is illustrated in this diagram.

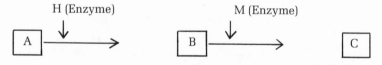

If there was a sequence of clinical reactions in the body necessary for normal functions: a substance A taken in the diet is broken up by a specific enzyme H into substance B; B is normally converted by a special enzyme M into a chemical product called C. If the disease was characterized by a missing enzyme M, then the chemical substance B cannot be broken down or digested by the body. Hence, substance B begins to accumulate excessively and is stored in organs like the liver, brain, eyes, or heart and begins to cause serious malfunctions in those organs, slowly or rapidly leading to death. One of the most recent and most exciting attempts at treatment has involved the delivery of the missing enzyme to the body. Hence the effort in the example shown in the diagram would be to provide either by mouth or directly into the blood the enzyme M, which would then get the process converting B to C working normally again. This unfortunately is easier said than done.

A whole host of problems that requires funding and research still exists for adequate progress to continue in this field. First, the technology to isolate and obtain the specific enzyme has to be further developed. The enzyme so derived has to be active, very stable, sterile, and made in such a way as not to stimulate the body to reject it. Each of those steps poses tremendous challenges.

Once the enzyme is obtained or isolated, some method of delivery into the body has to be devised. The most appropriate route is by mouth, but may not be possible for most enzymes because the acid in the stomach is apt to inactivate the enzyme. While much progress has been made in efforts to establish what we call enzyme therapy in hereditary disease, major obstacles remain to be overcome. Even if it were possible to administer the specific missing enzyme directly into the blood stream, the problem would be to ensure that the enzyme actually reaches and enters the tissue where the toxic products are accumulating. If that organ were the brain, the particular enzyme may simply not permeate the blood vessels into the brain cells where the real damage is occurring. This problem is proving to be a major obstacle, but if solved may one day allow for the option we all seek: to diagnose a genetic disease in the fetus and to initiate treatment in the womb.

Repair or Reconstruction

The development of a large head or hydrocephalus and associated mental retardation because of brain damage can be prevented by surgical techniques to decrease the pressure within the skull. Certain rerouting or shunting operations of major veins in the abdomen may be lifesaving in a few different kinds of hereditary disorders. Hereditary abnormalities of the face, the ears, the hands, feet, and so on, may all be remedied by "cosmetic" surgery. A defect may be passed down from one parent to half the children involving the lack of one or both ears. Through plastic surgery, it is possible to reconstruct a missing ear.

New Organs for Malfunctioning Ones

In hereditary diseases, it is unusual to have only a single organ affected. Yet it is possible, when a particular organ is especially damaged in the disease process, to remove and even replace it. Indeed, this technique has been applied to disabled kidneys, the implication being that kidney removal and transplantation of a new one will prevent further complications of the hereditary disease and allow the patient a more normal and possibly longer life. Some efforts have already been made in transplanting either the liver or spleen. Among the complex problems that arise with transplantation is not only the rejection of donated organs, but also the possibility that the hereditary disease may continue unabated and may even affect the donated organ.

There is sometimes a feeling of hopelessness when it comes to hereditary disease. The specific intent of this chapter was to provide just a brief insight into the many opportunities that exist for care and treatment, despite the absence of cure. Key to many of these approaches is the *early* initiation of treatment, which may prevent early death or irreversible mental retardation.

CHAPTER 23

Heredity, Intelligence, Race, and Learning Disorders

THROUGH PERSONAL EXPERIENCE, you may be aware of certain families rife with feeble-mindedness for generations. You may also have been puzzled to see remarkably brilliant individuals emerge from average or mediocre families. Is there really any way to correlate intelligence with heredity?

Definitions of intelligence are quite vague and refer, in essence, to "the ability to carry out abstract thinking." As early as 1905, I.Q. tests, as we know them today, were established mainly on the work of the French psychologist Alfred Binet. The tests he devised on behalf of the French Ministry of Education were specifically for measuring potential achievement in school. The American revisions of the Binet test were prepared initially at Stanford University, hence the name Stanford-Binet I.Q. Test.

Actual measurement of I.Q. is beset with a variety of problems. As currently applied, I.Q. tests are administered as a specific test in a specific way under specific conditions. They do attempt to measure a general intelligence factor, but fail in a number of ways. While they may indeed provide a fair measure of verbal, numerical, and inductive reasoning abilities, they fail to distinguish many other specific abilities (perhaps 120 in all!).

Many years ago, before revision, the Stanford-Binet test showed higher average I.Q.'s for boys than for girls. While there are those that might still believe that males have superior intellects, the facts are that careful revision of the test questions over many years now give almost identical I.Q. distributions for males and females. Although the test has been used as a measure of scholastic potential or success, it has fallen into disrepute because of its inability to account for the varying cultural, racial, or socioeconomic backgrounds of children in a mixed society. Hence, perfectly intelligent children from different cultural backgrounds may provide so-called wrong answers. A variety of tests have been developed to take care of these sociocultural biases, but none has yet fully achieved this goal. As far as whites are concerned, I.Q. tests do correlate very well with ultimate scholastic achievement. For other cultural backgrounds or ethnic groups, I.Q. tests must be viewed with considerable skepticism.

Some studies have shown that the I.Q. remains fairly constant between two and eighteen years of age. Other studies, in contrast, have showed changes of all sorts during the school years. Environmental factors that showed some effects were extreme parental permissiveness or extreme strictness, both being apparently responsible for decreases in I.Q. with increasing age.

Heredity and I.Q.

In 1906, well before the use of any kind of I.Q. test, some workers were concluding that 80 to 90 percent of intelligence is determined by heredity. Even Professor R. J. Herrnstein at Harvard came to a similar conclusion in 1971, as far as whites were concerned, after reviewing the history of intelligence testing. Professor Leon J. Kamin of Princeton University has written a perceptive analysis concerning the inheritability of I.Q. and concluded that virtually no good data exist that should make one accept any hypothesis suggesting that the I.Q. scores are in any degree inheritable. In the light of such contrasting views, what does the best evidence available show?

Twin Studies

We have referred many times in this book to the use of identical versus nonidentical twins in the assessment of inheritable characteristics. Since identical twins have identical genes, they provide a unique opportunity to study I.Q. But since they are reared together, the importance of environment may make interpretation of any study quite difficult. Hence, a number of different researchers elected to study identical twins who had been separated and reared apart. The expectations were that if heredity was of consequence in the development of I.Q., the scores achieved by parted identical twins should be extremely similar. As expected, some of the most extensive studies showed highly significant correlations between identical twins reared apart, suggesting a high degree of inheritability of I.Q.

Professor Kamin and others, however, have pointed to the fundamental fallacies of these studies. Besides the critically important technical and valid criticisms that he leveled at past studies of identical twins reared apart, he drew attention to the very similar environments in which these children were reared. In many instances in these studies, infants were placed in the homes of relatives or family friends. Hence, the effects of similar environment could have been confused with hereditary effects. He also suggested that the theoretical expectations of the person performing the test unconsciously bias the actual I.Q. measurement of twins. Furthermore, he noted that another possible source of bias depended upon the twins themselves providing detailed information about the extent of their separation. Kamin's conclusion from the separated identical twin studies is undoubtedly correct in that he concludes there are no adequate data to support the contention that I.Q. is simply inherited. This, of course, is not to say that hereditary factors make no contribution to the development of intelligence. The contrary is almost *certainly* true.

I.Q. Studies of Adopted Children

You may have thought that the practice of adoption would provide unique opportunities to determine the degree of hereditary influence on the development of intelligence. The adopted child, with genes from his biological parents, grows up in a new environment. If I.Q. was largely genetically determined, the adopted child's I.Q. should correlate closely with that of his true parents. So much for theory. In one large study, the average I.Q. of adopted children was 117, compared to the average I.Q. of their true mothers, which was 86! This large difference probably corresponds to significant differences in the socioeconomic status of the adopting families. Obviously, adopted children are very often placed in homes that are more advantageous than those of the biological parents. The environmental effects on those living in a "selected" family are not negligible.

In another study, the correlation of I.Q. of the adopted parents with their own children was even slightly lower than was the correlation with their adopted children! This would suggest no effect of genes at all! The opposite has also been found. Certainly expectations that studies of adopted children would clarify the importance of hereditary influences have not as yet been realized. The innumerable factors that impinge upon the development of intelligence make it difficult to come to solid conclusions about the relative effects of environment and heredity.

Factors Influencing the Development and Measurement of I.Q.

Family Factors

Studies in Scotland, France, the Netherlands, and the United States on children between six and nineteen years of age all indicate that the intellectual level generally declines as family size increases. While it is known that family size differs across the strata of society, the studies just referred to revealed that I.Q. declined with increased family size *independently* of status, though it goes without saying that socioeconomic conditions affect I.Q. scores.

American and Dutch studies furthermore show that I.Q. also declines with birth order. That is to say the I.Q.'s of children born toward the end of a large family are generally lower than those of the first few children in the family. One further dimension to this question of birth order is the spacing of children within families. There appears to be a relationship between the general decline of I.Q. with birth order when the intervals between children are especially short.

Single parent homes are more likely to constitute inferior intellectual environments, which should be reflected in generally lower intellectual abilities in the children of such homes. Early loss of one parent would be expected similarly to produce an intellectually suboptimal environment than a parental loss at a later age. In both these instances, studies have indeed come to these conclusions. One study, for example, showed that fatherless students scored significantly lower in the American college entrance examination test compared with children from intact homes. Indeed, differences in intellectual performance found between children from fatherless homes and from intact homes have been found to be greater the earlier the father's death or departure and the younger the child when parental absence began. Death, divorce, or separation is also invariably associated with emotional chaos or stress in the home, which again, as expected, is associated with diminished intellectual performance. Such intellectual deficits have been found to occur even when the father's absence is temporary and where there is no significant stressful situation because of his absence. The return of the missing adult has clearly been shown to be beneficial. For example, the remarriage of the remaining parent of a young child has been shown to result in the improved intellectual performance of that child.

Besides the peculiarities of the administered I.Q. tests in reflecting differences between the sexes, other hidden factors may also be affecting these assessments. For example, intervals following male births appear to be somewhat longer than those following female births (possibly because of parental preference for male children). Females are found more frequently later in the family than are males. Finally, it has been known for many years that more fetal and newborn deaths occur among males than among females. Fetal deaths also occur with a higher frequency in older mothers. All these factors could therefore combine to produce sex differences as reflected by I.Q. tests.

Twins and I.Q.

Twins are known to score consistently and substantially lower on I.Q. tests and other tests of intellectual performance than other children. Not unexpectedly, triplets (in general) score lower than twins. Probably the most important factor explaining these differences is the birth weight of twins, which is invariably lower than in non-twins. The higher frequency of prematurity, the associated complications due to lack of oxygen, hypoglycemia (low blood sugar), jaundice, and other complications constitute adverse factors in the development of intellectual function. Although that sounds sufficient as an explanation, it is not the whole story.

You would expect that the intellectual performance of twins who were separated earlier in life should be higher than that of twins reared together (because of more individual attention and care per hour per child). The importance of environmental effects on the development of intellectual growth of twins is reflected in a report showing that twins whose co-twins were stillborn or died within four weeks achieved nearly the same I.Q.'s as non-twins! Low birth weight and its associated complications in twins are clearly not the only explanations for why twins usually do less well than others.

Race and I.Q.

You are undoubtedly aware of the extensive public discussion and controversy that have centered in recent years on the relationship of I.Q. to race. That discussion has mainly sought to explain why the I.Q.'s of blacks, in particular, have generally been found to be lower than whites. There are those very vocal scientists who have tried unconvincingly to maintain that blacks are genetically inferior to whites. Perhaps the absurdity of any such claim is already obvious to you in the light of the aforegoing discussion. Perhaps a brief summary of the issues that impinge on the I.Q. and race question would be useful.

The difference in I.Q. scores between blacks and whites in the United States has been found to be of the order of 15 I.Q. points. You recall we referred to the fact that there is, at present, no truly culture-free I.Q. test, and that available tests can hardly be considered an assessment of innate ability, simply because they depend on development having taken place against a specific cultural background. Those scholars claiming a genetic basis to explain the differences in I.Q.'s between blacks and whites have essentially failed to consider fully the extent of environmental influences on the development of I.Q. We have referred above to most of the factors that would adversely affect the development of I.Q. in blacks. Their generally lower socioeconomic status, poorer nutrition, more frequent parental absence, higher frequency of low birth weight and prematurity, larger family sizes, shorter spacing between children, the associated sociocultural deprivation, the decreased educational opportunities, and so many other factors all unequivocally make more blacks than whites socially disadvantaged. The consequences for I.Q. development should be obvious. Moreover, being black may also carry with it a social burden not suffered by whites. The role of chronic though low grade lead poisoning — a plight of poor urban black (and white) communities in the United States — cannot be ignored either.

Of additional interest is that the I.Q.'s of children born to older mothers are consistently higher than those born to younger mothers. Hence, it may be significant that white mothers in the United States are on the average nearly three years older at the birth of their first child than are black mothers.

If, indeed, there were genetic differences between blacks and whites as far as I.Q. was concerned, such an argument should be supported by differences observed between black and white children raised in the same environment. A study in England compared black, white, and mixed parentage children and revealed no significant differences between the groups, although white children tended to have the lowest average scores of three tests.

In another study, an attempt was made to correlate the I.Q. of American blacks with their probable degree of white ancestry as judged by blood group similarities. The data tended to show that the I.Q. of blacks seemed to be lowered by white ancestry, but the results were not statistically significant.

Just as for stature, it is likely that the quality of intelligence is inherited to some extent. That any individual's final abilities reflect interaction between genetic endowment and environment should be obvious to all. Equally obvious, perhaps, is the counterproductive and incorrect conclusions that make efforts to suggest the inferiority of one race to another simply on the basis of a questionably valid I.Q. test.

Learning Disorders

Brain damage or dysfunction may lead to learning disabilities. The first obvious type is when the brain has been damaged during birth, for example, by lack of oxygen or by hemorrhage, resulting in varying degrees of brain dysfunction, and is associated with other signs of brain damage, such as spastic limbs or inability to speak. A second, though not so obvious, type of brain dysfunction is suspected to be the result of damage to certain areas of the brain in the fetus causing disabilities in the development of language, speech, hearing, as well as abnormal body movement, as in the hyperkinetic child. This syndrome is frequently referred to as minimal brain dysfunction. In actuality, no characteristic brain damage has been discovered in those affected children.

The third type of brain dysfunction results probably from hereditary influences that interfere with the development of perceptual function including the ability to read and the acquisition of language. This is the group in which we recognize dyslexia, which, by the way, is derived from Greek and simply means reading disorder. Of all the known learning disabilities, the best information about hereditary aspects, though incomplete, refers to dyslexia, to which we will confine our considerations. The term *learning disability* refers to those disorders involved in understanding or using language, spoken or written, which may manifest as an imperfect ability to listen, think, speak, read, write, spell, or do math.

Dyslexia is an extremely common condition being found in some one or two out of every ten adults in Western countries, that is, about 15 percent of the population. Again, we are referring specifically to reading disability that persists into adult life and may be associated with handwriting problems:

reversals and rotations of letters as well as additions, deletions, or substitutions of letters. Three further essential characteristics of dyslexia are that the disability exists *despite* adequate intelligence, without sociocultural deprivation, and in the absence of any other obvious brain disorder.

Parents and doctors alike know that children with learning disorders frequently have behavioral or emotional difficulties. On occasion, the question is raised whether these difficulties are a cause or a consequence of the learning disorder. It is also well recognized that children with learning disorders not infrequently come from chaotic home environments or from families with serious problems; therefore, it is sometimes difficult to distinguish environment from heredity as the prime cause. Obviously, it is important to distinguish the hereditary aspects, since if a problem can be anticipated, early remedies may successfully be sought. Under favorable conditions, most children with dyslexia can be taught to read and spell so as to be fully capable of pursuing any career of their choice.

Hereditary Aspects of Dyslexia

As long ago as 1905, evidence suggested that dyslexia tended to occur within families. One of the most careful and important studies on its genetic aspects was done by Dr. B. Hallgren on children attending the Stockholm Child Guidance Clinic in Sweden. Some 276 patients were carefully evaluated, all but six of the children being personally examined by Dr. Hallgren. He observed that 88 percent had a family history of one or more members with reading problems. From a genetic point of view, the conclusion was that dyslexia was transmitted as a dominant disorder. That is, an affected parent would pass along the gene for dyslexia to 50 percent of his or her children. Further Scandinavian studies at the same center focused on twins with dyslexia. In each case studied, twins who were identical both had dyslexia, which in genetic terminology is described as 100 percent concordance. For the nonidentical twins, only one in three pairs was found where both members had the disorder. Other studies have come to similar conclusions.

Dyslexia affects males much more often than females; Dr. MacDonald Critchley in London calculated that out of his enormous experience, there were four males with dyslexia for each female so afflicted. In the Scandinavian studies, marriage between first cousins or other close relatives was not found to be a consequential factor in the genetic aspects of this disorder.

It would seem highly likely that there is more than one hereditary type of dyslexia, the most important being the dominant form already referred to above. One could therefore expect in certain families that one of the parents may have the disorder in an extremely mild form — perhaps barely detectable. Many dominant diseases are due to mutation, and this would explain isolated cases within a family, a single gene mutation being responsible. In such cases, with both parents normal, the risk of having another dyslexic child would be zero, in contrast to the situation where one parent is clearly affected, with a 50 percent risk of passing it on to each subsequent child. It is also possible with dominant inheritance (see Chapter 5) for the disorder to involve one sex especially.

Another likely form of inheritance is via the X chromosome of the mother, as in hemophilia and muscular dystrophy. The mother might be the carrier of the dyslexia gene, with a risk of 50 percent of her sons being affected and 50 percent of her daughters being carriers.

More still needs to be done on the genetics of dyslexia. Analysis and evaluation of hereditary patterns have been confounded because many individuals have different combinations of disabilities, such as speech problems together with dyslexia.

The Hyperkinetic Child Syndrome

This condition was described by a German physician over 100 years ago. Its main features include varying degrees of hyperactivity and easy distractibility. The children tend to be very impulsive and excitable as well as antisocial in behavior. A whole range of other emotional and behavioral symptoms is also seen in hyperactive children. This disorder is thought to be quite common, affecting in its most florid form perhaps a few percent of all school-age populations. Again, as for dyslexia, boys predominate by far, the boy/girl ratio varying between 4 to 1 and 9 to 1.

It has long been suspected that the problem of hyperactive children is a familial one. As usual, the major problem has been the inability to separate out environmental effects from genetic endowment. For example, Dr. Dennis P. Cantwell, in California, and other researchers have shown that between one-third and one-half of the parents of such children have some psychiatric problem. A greater prevalence of alcoholism, psychopathic disorders, and hysteria has been observed in the parents of hyperactive children than in matched populations studied together.

Adopted children have been studied to determine the frequency of hyperactivity. In the reported studies, the hyperactive child syndrome was found much more frequently in the true relatives of the adopted child, pointing to hereditary factors. Studies of identical and nonidentical twins have also shown a greater frequency of both identical twins being affected compared to the rate noted in nonidentical twins.

The little evidence there is clearly implies *some* hereditary factors, but the interaction here between inheritance and conditioning is so complicated that no reliable statement can be offered. If you have one child with this disorder, there is no sure way of predicting the likelihood of this syndrome happening again.

Hereditary Disorders and High I.Q.

It has been known for some time that superior intelligence has been associated with a number of different hereditary disorders. In one condition called torsion dystonia, the affected person has dreadful muscle spasms, is unable to walk or eat without aid, and is generally totally incapacitated yet exhibits great intelligence. People affected by the hereditary eye tumor (retinoblastoma) have also been observed to have high

I.Q.'s. In some individuals whose blood uric acid is high, a condition called hyperuricemia, questions have arisen whether the higher I.Q. levels they exhibit are apt to be due to the uric acid stimulating the brain. Brothers and sisters of patients with phenylketonuria have also been found to have above average intelligence. A similar observation has been made about the parents of autistic children.

Recently, some compelling evidence has arisen in studies in California on nearsighted young people. Studies were done on 2527 high-school students aged seventeen to eighteen years, of whom 377 were nearsighted (myopic). Their I.Q.'s had been tested about ten years before, even before most had realized that they were, in fact, nearsighted. The results showed that at age seventeen to eighteen those youngsters who were nearsighted scored higher I.Q.'s than their peers. The frequency of nearsightedness was highest amongst those students who had the highest I.Q.'s. Looking back, the researchers noted high I.Q. levels ten years earlier in those who subsequently developed nearsightedness! So the bespectacled individual may not only look bright, but often is.

CHAPTER 24

Do Your Genes Determine
How Long You Will Live?

WHY, YOU MAY ASK, do we all die? We understand why
death occurs when a person has cancer, heart disease, high
blood pressure, stroke, or some other disease or disorder. But
if no disease confounds our efforts to live on and on, why
don't we? Do we all simply just wear out? Why do females
live longer than males? This, in fact, is not confined to the
human species, since female spiders, fish, water beetles, house
flies, chickens, and fruit flies all live longer than their male
counterparts. (Yet there *are* some birds, especially pigeons,
where the males reputedly live longer than females.)
Strangely, in humans, more male than female newborn babies
die.

Lessons about Aging from Animals?

It would seem that specifically circumscribed lifespans are
equally characteristic in the animal kingdom, as is the case for
the human. The lifespan of the mouse rarely exceeds two
years, rats four years, cats thirty years, elephants sixty years,
and horses forty years.

Experimentally, rats that have been fed diets that were sufficient in all constituents except calories showed growth retardation during the period of calorie restriction. After increasing the calorie intake, the rats proceeded to grow to adult size
and eventually exceeded the normal expected lifespan for that
strain of rats. They reached about twice the maximum age
achieved by rats whose diets were not interdicted. Similar
results have been noted in chickens, bees, silkworms, and
other species. The effects on prolonging life were most pronounced when low calorie diets were started soon after birth.
Of particular interest was the observation that those rats who

were initially on the calorie restricted diet had an associated delay of onset of various tumors and chronic diseases related to aging.

Even the surrounding temperature in which we live has been questioned in its relationship to age. Fish raised at low temperatures have better growth and live longer. Rats, on the other hand, when reared at low room temperatures, have a considerable decrease in their lifespan from all causes of death, including for some strange reason, cancer!

Removal of the sex glands of salmon early in their development has been noted to prolong their lifespan.

Mice raised in a germ-free environment have been shown to have a longer mean lifespan, as have rats who have had their spleens removed early in life. The implication of both of these experiments is that the body defenses active against infection (called autoimmune mechanisms) may clearly be implicated in the aging process.

The implication of different longevity in males and females mentioned above suggests the influence of the sex hormones. In this context, therefore, it is interesting to note that among cats, those who have been castrated have attained the highest recorded ages. No equivalent human data exist. Some female fruit flies that are virgins, born without ovaries, or are sterilized live longer than their normal female contemporaries. While virgin mice live longer than spayed females, the oldest of all are castrated mice.

The Death Clocks

The death of cells is a normal accompaniment to development in animals. Indeed, whole tissues or organs are constantly being destroyed. This is the mechanism by which organs, useful only during the larval or embryonic stages of many animals, are eliminated. Degeneration and death of cells is crucial, too, in the development of limbs in certain animals, especially in modeling not only digits, but also the contours of whole limbs. Cell death is an intrinsic part of normal animal development.

If there were a clear genetic effect on aging, then it should be evident in studying identical twins. After all, identical twins, as we all know, originate from a single fertilized egg, whereas nonidentical twins develop from two eggs. Any differences noted between identical twins, as discussed earlier, must be a reflection of environmental influences. Identical twins, on average, appear to die within five years of each other, although a much greater spread does occur in individual cases. Nonidentical twins die much farther apart. It is interesting that male twins generally have shorter lifespans than female twins.

Centenarians

Professor Alexander Leaf of the Massachusetts General Hospital traveled to the Russian Caucasus to study certain aspects of aging in that population. In the Caucasus according to a 1970 census, there are apparently some 5000 centenarians or persons who have reached at least 100 years of age. Many live in the Soviet republic of Georgia. The reason for their aggregation there is uncertain. Very many live at high altitudes above the sea (1500 to 4500 feet). Industrial centers appear to have the lowest percentage of centenarians. We do not know whether pollution, urban stress, and other factors hasten the aging process or not.

Even in Soviet Georgia there is a preponderance, about two-thirds, of females over the age of ninety. A similar preponderance of surviving females over males is evident in the United States. The difficulties of documenting exact ages in persons over 100 years in Russia and elsewhere are acknowledged by all authorities. A Russian male, who died in 1973, claimed to be 168 years old. The 1975 edition of the *Guinness Book of World Records* holds that the longest documented human life was 113 years, 124 days; that centenarian male was a French-Canadian bootmaker.

Why Do We Age?

The exact reason is really not understood. Married men appear to live longer than unmarried men. I am sure you can think of a hundred reasons why this should be so. More or less sexual activity may be one of the thoughts that crossed your mind? Certainly, it is established in rats that old males live appreciably longer if a young female is provided to groom them. A number of studies have demonstrated that children of long-lived parents have a longer lifespan compared to the offspring of short-lived parents, though the difference is unimpressive.

Not too much has been spent on aging research. In 1972, the United States government spent only about four cents per person on it, compared to the two dollars per person for cancer research and about one dollar per person for heart and lung research. In California, attention has been drawn to the point that cures for both cancer and heart disease would increase human life expectancy only by about nine years and would not change our total lifespan. Calls for the funding of concentrated efforts to increase our life expectancy have therefore rightly been made. Meanwhile, we are still beset with theories or hypotheses about why we get old.

Your Cells Are Programmed by Your Genes

Perhaps the most accepted theory of aging suggests that the blueprint for your total lifespan is "written in your genes," and is apparent from the moment you are conceived. The basis for this information is fascinating.

If you took a tiny pinch of skin and grew it in tissue culture in the laboratory, you would discover that its cells have a fairly fixed lifespan. These cells or fibroblasts have been grown from many persons. We know that each cell is able to grow and double itself about 40 to 60 times over. After that it simply dies. The same studies have been done for different animal species, and the same limited lifespan of cells has been demonstrated. Moreover, it appears that the lifetime of each cell is directly proportional to the average lifespan of that species. Hence, for men and women, these fibroblast cells on average double about 50 times before dying and relate to the usual human lifespan of about seventy years. Cells from the chicken, in contrast, double some 15 to 35 times, which is directly related to the average maximum lifespan of thirty years. The evidence indicates that the number of times a cell can divide is fixed in our inborn genetic messages.

One could take these fibroblast cells from any species including man and freeze them at minus 196°C in liquid nitrogen. Although kept in storage for months or many years, when thawed they can be grown again. They simply resume dividing and doubling just where they left off! Their "memory" is clear and accurate: probably "programmed" in the genes.

Cells grown from tiny pieces of skin taken from an old person are found to have curtailed lifespans when compared with cells taken from infants. Again the implication is that for each of us aging is basically fixed from the start by "aging genes" that program our cells for a certain span, at the end of which time they cease to function normally, senile changes occur, and eventually we die. This theory is fortified by the inevitability of the menopause. Completely predictable, its exact timing is probably influenced or controlled by heredity, just as, some say, is aging.

Or the Machine Simply Breaks Down

Another theory holds that there are no specific aging genes, but, rather, that our cells, in the course of living, dividing, and growing, are subject to environmental influences as well as to biochemical changes, as time goes on. The idea is that molecules within the cell become damaged in some way, causing breakdowns in the cell machinery and subsequent errors in function. The precise nature of this sort of damage is really not understood, but it is known that such errors or changes, which may be mutations, do occur. Possibly the known repair systems our cells contain become inefficient or defective. Ultimately, accumulated errors and changes could cause sufficiently dangerous malfunction to lead to cell and then body death.

External environment, however, cannot be underestimated. During the Second World War, studies performed during the development of atomic energy showed that various forms of x-rays, when given in sublethal doses to young animals, such as mice, caused them to die of "old age" earlier than their contemporaries. The x-rayed animals not only looked older, but also died earlier of the same diseases their nonirradiated litter mates had.

It is certainly conceivable that agents such as x-rays have an adverse effect on human longevity.

Aging Due to Infection?

Study of both animals and humans clearly shows that viruses may persist in tissues throughout life in spite of the continuous effort of the body to fight them with antibodies. As a matter of fact, the battle between antibodies and the invading virus may injure the cells and bring on degenerative diseases, such as presenile dementia, in adult life. Though it is more reasonable to assume that aging results from multiple factors, it is possible to imagine that viruses by persisting in cells may lead to or enhance their malfunction and thereby influence the rate of growing old.

Premature Aging

It can no longer be disputed that some hereditary defects can bring old age on sooner, though the mechanism is still to be discovered. One distressing, rare condition is called progeria. It is characterized by an aging process so accelerated that children who have it resemble old people before they are ten years of age. They have stunted growth and serious disease of all the major blood vessels including the coronaries; they may become bald and are often thin and wrinkled. Death comes early, almost always before twenty, usually from heart disease or pneumonia. All the evidence we have suggests that both parents of such an afflicted child are carriers of the gene, but the mechanism behind this tragic condition is unknown.

Another premature aging disorder is called Werner's syndrome, probably transmitted in the same way as progeria, by two parents who are carriers. The victims have stunted growth, develop cataracts early in life, become gray or actually bald, and tend to develop diabetes as well as major disease of the blood vessels. Moreover, their bones become less dense (this is called osteoporosis), and there is a high frequency of cancer. Again, the causative mechanism is totally obscure.

As for normal aging, we can only conjecture. The die may be cast the moment we are conceived; that single cell that comes into being when the sperm fuses with the egg may contain the blueprint — the plan — of a life that will last, if not cut off by disease or accident, for sixty-eight years. Or ninety years. And so on. Or it may be environment that precipitates aging. You must have heard of or even seen a person "age overnight" because of some personal tragedy. Does the mind have some psychic influence over the aging process?

Whatever the cause — and it is likely to be *causes* — the whole matter is extremely complex and far from resolution.

CHAPTER 25

Predicting or Choosing the Sex of Your Baby

THROUGHOUT RECORDED HISTORY, people have tried to predict the sex of a coming child. All manner of magic has been evoked: astrology, numerology, dreams, examination of the entrails of sacrificed animals, the pattern of flights of birds, and the use of other supernatural techniques. The political importance of producing a male child has dominated society — from royalty down to those who till the soil. Not surprisingly, world literature is replete with descriptions of how to tell if a girl or a boy will be born.

Predictions of the Past

The Answer Was in the Barley

Perhaps the oldest of these recorded methods is to be found in Egyptian papyri dated around 1350 B.C.E. describing a technique that combined the diagnosis of pregnancy with a prediction of fetal sex. This system required the urine of the woman, which was used to moisten daily samples of barley and wheat. If the barley was found to be germinating, a female would be born. If the wheat was found to be germinating, a male. If no germination occurred, the woman was not pregnant. Some research workers in 1933 experimented with this ancient technique. They reported a correct prediction in 80 percent of the cases!

Facial Color

From the Egyptian papyri we learn that the sex of the fetus could also be predicted from the color of the pregnant woman's face. If, for example, the face had a greenish hue, a male was virtually certain to be born. In Hippocrates' time, it was thought that a woman with a male fetus had a "good color" but a poor facial color if the fetus was a female. Aristotle chauvinistically maintained that females have a lower developmental level than males and, consequently, a male fetus makes more demands on the mother than the female fetus, thereby needing greater body warmth and better circulation.

Moods, Dreams, and Beliefs

The mood of the pregnant woman appears also to be important in the prediction of fetal sex. A male fetus is likely if the mother is cheerful, according to the Arabian belief; if happy, according to the Indian belief; and if untroubled, according to Jewish belief.

Interpreters of dreams in India have held that if the woman dreams about men's food, then she must be carrying a male. In Russia, dreams of knives or clubs spell a male baby in contrast to dreams about spring or about parties that clearly denote a female.

During the tenth century in Japan, it was thought that women desiring a boy should concentrate on male activities, such as hunting. While not wanting to stretch your credulity too far, would you believe that until recent times, the Japanese believed that if a husband called to his wife while she was on her way to the toilet, and caused her to turn suddenly to the left, a female would be born. The idea was, no doubt, that the right side of the body, always considered to be the stronger and more valuable side, was male, and vice versa. Both in the sixth and eleventh centuries, there was a belief that the breasts should be watched closely in early pregnancy, since in the presence of a male fetus, the right breast would be larger and secrete milk earlier with the right areola (colored area around the nipple) larger and darker with a redder, more projecting nipple. Many other methods of prediction had to do with the power of the right side in one way or another. One curious one was that salt would not melt on the right nipple if a male was being carried!

A variety of ideas have existed from time to time concerning both the activities and position of the fetus. As expected, some have believed that the male fetus not only moves earlier, but kicks harder — and, of course, mainly on the right side. In Sweden, it was believed that the spreading of the rear end suggested that the pregnant woman was carrying a female, while the reverse was believed in France. Some have believed that the pigment that may be deposited in the midline, between the pubic hairline and the navel, if dark signifies a male fetus. The appearance of freckles on a woman's face often meant the presence of a male fetus, although some believed the opposite. Excessive vomiting can imply to some that the woman is carrying a male fetus. Even the quality of the breast milk has been used for sex prediction. If a boy, the milk, especially from the right breast, was expected to be thick and viscous. Or, if some of this milk was dropped into water and fell to the bottom, a male was predicted. If, however, it floated on the surface or even dissolved, then a baby of the "weaker sex" would be born.

Sex and the Father

The role of the father in determining the sex of the future child was not entirely ignored. One idea was that if the male in coitus had tied up the *left* testicle, then he would of course have male offspring. As late as the eighteenth century, French noblemen who wished to have a male heir were told that removal of the left testicle would assure them of that result.

Modern Methods of Sex Determination

The fetal sex can be determined today by staining cells derived from the fetus and found floating in the amniotic fluid. What is even more accurate is the determination of the chromosomal pattern that is possible by study of the growing amniotic cells in the laboratory (see Chapters 14 and 15). Other methods, such as using cells in the mucus from the cervix, have *not* proved to be consistent or reliable in sex determination. The most pressing reasons nowadays to determine the fetal sex are related to the risk of having a child with a hereditary disease confined to males only (see Chapter 5). There are also a few very rare disorders — transmitted in a different way than the sex-linked disorders — that cause the parents to elect to have only males.

The use of amniocentesis and prenatal genetic studies simply for family planning purposes is, at present, as I have said, a most inappropriate use of a very scarce and expensive technology. Moreover, there is a certain repugnance shared by many for a process that aims to abort a pregnancy simply on the basis of individual family sex preferences.

Selecting the Sex of Your Future Child

A more rational approach to family planning that allows selection of the sex of your children in order to avoid recurrence of a hereditary disease or defect has been heralded by new and exciting progress in medical genetics. It became possible around 1970, by using a simple staining technique, to show that about half of all sperm bear a Y chromosome (and would therefore make a male) and half the sperm bear an X chromosome (and would therefore make a female).

In 1973, more progress was made in separating out male-determining from female-determining sperms. The techniques utilized were based upon prior knowledge that the former have a superior swimming ability compared to the female-determining sperm. This apparently reliable technique allows for the separation of 85 percent of swimming (and, presumably, functional) male-determining sperms. The female-determining sperms, or the X-bearing sperms, are heavier and therefore slower, since they contain up to 4 percent more genetic material (DNA) than the Y male-bearing sperm. It would seem to be virtually certain that isolation of male- from female-determining sperm samples will be achieved in the near future. The pleasure of purposeful procreation would then be lost, of course, since the samples of the husband's semen would have to be worked on and the wife then artificially inseminated!

Success with the technique would therefore obviate the need for consideration of abortion for all those couples facing risks of offspring with sex-linked diseases, for example, hemophilia or muscular dystrophy. Such couples could then choose simply to have female offspring. Moreover, those couples who desire to select the sex of their children for less drastic reasons could also do so without the need to resort to abortion because the "unwanted sex" was found in the fetus.

Meanwhile, Back at the Ranch!

Medical technological breakthroughs tend to take time. Until the technique just described is perfected, information currently available might help you in trying to select the sex of your children:

Ovulation usually occurs 12 to 16 days *before* the beginning of the next menstrual period. The egg can be fertilized for some 6 to 24 hours after ovulation. The sperm is able to achieve fertilization for 24 to 48 hours after intercourse or artificial insemination.

A variety of factors may influence fertilization occurring by an X-bearing (female) or Y-bearing (male) sperm. The acidity or alkalinity of the vaginal (and cervical) secretions may be important. The woman's body temperature usually rises at ovulation, and this, too, may affect the two different types of sperm. The age of the sperm may be relevant. The less frequently coitus occurs, the "older" the sperm, and it seems the more likely that males will be conceived. During the Second World War, in both England and the United States, appreciably more males than females were born, perhaps bearing out the theory.

The best information, today, points to a great likelihood of having males if coitus occurs four or more days before the woman's temperature rises, or one or more days thereafter. The *opposite* has been noted following artificial insemination.

Some Implications of Preselecting the Sex of Your Children

The ratio of the two sexes at birth is not quite as equally distributed as might be expected. There is in fact a slight excess of males, which led a distinguished biologist some years ago to remark that we were heading for a world shortage of marriageable females. Most evidence currently indicates that if couples were offered the opportunity to select the sex of their children, the result would be an increased proportion of males in the population. Undoubtedly, different social classes and ethnic groups would have different preferences. It is extremely likely that in less developed countries male children would still seem to be a more positive acquisition to a family as a help in working the land, earning money for food, performing necessary rites at the graves of their parents and ancestors, and so on.

In a recent study involving 100 pregnant women, a female fetus was detected in 46. Some 29 of these women elected to abort simply for that reason Only 1 woman out of the 53 found to be carrying a male fetus chose to abort. (In one of the cases, the fetal sex was not determined.) The study was done in China, at the Tietung Hospital of Anshan Iron and Steel Company. Its aim was to assist in family planning.

Many parents appear to desire one of each sex. The opportunity of being able to choose the sex of one's children might ultimately reduce both family size and the population, since couples with children of the same sex are more likely to have additional children than are couples who have achieved both a boy and a girl. A similar tendency has also been noted: that women who have had only daughters have more children than those with only sons. Information available clearly documents that today, as throughout history, couples have consistent preferences for male offspring and tend to prefer a boy to be the firstborn.

If sex preselection does become routinely available, certain ominous predictions have been made in the light of this recognized preference. Professor Amitai Etzioni of Columbia University predicted in 1968 that an excess of males in the population would lead to an increase in prostitution, homosexuality, marriage between males, and an increase in the number of males who never marry.

You might assume that most parents, given the opportunity of preselecting the sex of their child, would avail themselves of it. But current attitudes of married women in the United States indicate that many would not wish to be able to choose the sex of their children. These attitudes may well be modified, however, when the technology does become available and socially acceptable.

CHAPTER 26

Twins

TWINS, even in today's matter-of-fact world, still invariably evoke comment, whether it be at the news of their birth, on the street, in school, and so on. At least, nowadays, the birth of twins is not regarded as a threat to society, as was the case not so many years ago. Various taboos arose from fear and ignorance of what was then considered an uncanny event.

During medieval times and earlier, the mother and her twins were reviled in many countries, since she was thought to have been unfaithful and each twin had been sired by a different father or by an evil spirit. Mythology is replete with horrors in which both children were killed, or at least one, and frequently the mother as well. (One idea is that the revulsion stemmed from identification of twins with the multiple births of animals.) You may recall that the twins Romulus and Remus, born in ancient Rome, were destined to die with their mother.

Interest in our scientific age has focused rather on the mechanism and causes of twinning. The purpose in this chapter is to provide you with an insight into these causes that, as usual, seem to be an intertwining of influences with genetic predisposition.

Types of Twins

Identical twins arise from a single fertilized egg that divides into two separate embryos within 14 days after fertilization. Fraternal or nonidentical twins originate from the fertilization of two different eggs, usually at the same time. In at least one documented case studied with blood groups, fertilization of two eggs occurred a month apart and was caused by two men. The "twins" were, therefore, allegedly one month different in age. This case stretches the imagination somewhat, and confirmation of such an occurrence is awaited with obvious interest.

How Frequently Do Multiple Births Occur?

Nonidentical twins are born at different rates in various parts of the world. Rates are high in Africa, low in the Far East, and intermediate in the United States, Europe, and India. In the United States, Britain, and Europe about 1 in 80 pregnancies in whites concludes with twins, the rate being somewhat higher in blacks. The highest rates reported are from tribes in western Nigeria, where close to 1 in 25 births are twins.

Triplets occur somewhere between 1 in 5,000 and 1 in 10,000 births. Quadruplets were thought to occur about once in 500,000 births, and quintuplets once in 50 million births. The use of the new fertility drugs has clearly increased the frequency of these multiple births in the last few years. The first quintuplets who lived to attain adult age were born in Canada in 1934 — the Dionne sisters. Many other sets have now been reported from all over the world. One elegantly studied case involved quintuplets born in Danzig, Poland. Their blood groups showed that they each arose from a different fertilized egg.

The Causes of Twinning

A variety of possible influences may induce twinning to occur. The matter is complex and can possibly best be considered under two familiar headings: environmental and genetic.

Environmental Influences   Identical twins are born at about the same rate all over the world, and factors such as race, the age of the mother, or nutrition do not appear to influence that rate. The exact cause leading a fertilized egg to split into two embryos is unknown, and seems to be a random phenomenon, but may be related to certain environmental factors, or a transient lack of oxygen to the embryo.

In contrast, a variety of environmental factors seem to be operating in nonidentical twinning. In Finland, for example, the frequency of twin births is highest in July and lowest in January. This observation prompted the suggestion that the long exposure to sunlight in the Finnish summer stimulates hormone production resulting in the release of more than one egg at a time. One study in the state of New York, however, failed to show any seasonal difference in the rate of twinning.

The likelihood of twins appears to be greater when women become pregnant within the first three months after marriage. Interestingly, stress or impaired nutrition may decrease the likelihood only of nonidentical twin births, as was noted during the Second World War.

It is well recognized that an increased frequency (as much as fivefold) of nonidentical twins occurs with increasing age of the mother, reaching a peak between thirty-five and thirty-nine years, the frequency dropping off rapidly thereafter. Moreover, the more children a woman has, the more likely she is to have nonidentical twins. Some workers have noted that the chances of having twins increase with the height of the mother; the taller the mother, the greater the chances. Also, obese women appear to have a greater likelihood of having nonidentical twins than thin women. Finally, and wholly unexplained, is the observation that twins occur more often in illegitimate pregnancies compared with the rate in the general population.

A Genetic Predisposition to Have Twins? Throughout this book, I have referred repeatedly to studies of twins for different diseases. The idea has been that identical twins share identical genes and should therefore be subject to the same diseases — if *hereditary* — in contrast to nonidentical twins. A genetic predisposition to have *nonidentical* twins is, however, a different matter. It should already be clear to you that having *identical* twins does not appear to be influenced by genetic mechanisms or family history.

Most of us have heard of families where nonidentical twin births have appeared in successive generations. There certainly are some remarkable examples reported in the medical literature. There is the reputed case of a Dr. Mary Austin who, during 33 years of marriage, apparently had 44 children: 13 pairs of twins and 6 sets of triplets. It was said, in 1896, that one of her sisters had given birth to 26 children, and another sister to 41 children. An unusual case is reported of an American fisherman, whose wife gave birth to their first pair of twins in October, 1945. The couple subsequently had a second pair of twins in October of the following year and a third pair of twins again in October of the year after that. This gave them a total of six children in three years. In 1938, a woman was noted to have given birth to six pairs of nonidentical twins, between whom were interspersed some single births. This woman's father had a set of triplets with his second wife. In another remarkable case reported in 1918, a woman had triplets in her first pregnancy and delivered a second set of triplets in her second pregnancy nine months later. She had six sons in one year. (The Internal Revenue Service should have paid *her* that year!)

In certain families, the father has been attributed as being important in transmitting the tendency. A celebrated case turned up in 1914 concerning a Russian peasant who married twice. It was said that his first wife gave birth to four sets of quadruplets, seven sets of triplets, and sixteen pairs of twins. Clearly inexhaustible, he married again and with his second wife had two sets of triplets and six pairs of twins. This gentleman, therefore, had a grand total of 87 children, 84 of whom survived.

Again, supporting possible hereditary factors in the male was the reported case of a man who, himself a twin, had nine pairs of twins with his first wife. His wife remarried and subsequently gave birth to six single sons.

Except for these very unusual families, the father generally does not appear to have a significant role in the frequency of twinning. If anything, the best available data imply that the role of the mother is much more important. Studies based on the excellent family records of the Mormon Church of Salt

Lake City, Utah, showed that women who were themselves nonidentical twins and their sisters had twins much more often than did the general population. Men who were themselves nonidentical twins and their brothers did not have twins more often than others in the community. Other studies have borne out these conclusions. Most recent evidence shows that mothers who have *identical* twins do not have a higher likelihood of repeating such births; but mothers of *nonidentical* twins appear to have about twice as high a chance as normal of having another twin birth.

The exact reason or mechanism explaining why certain women are more predisposed to having nonidentical twins is not known. Perhaps the most important postulate — and one supported by data — is that a higher level of certain sex hormones (from the pituitary gland) is found in the blood of these women. These hormones might facilitate double ovulation, and the control of their secretions may be genetically determined and transmitted through the women of the family. This is still conjectural.

Birth Defects in Twins

A high rate of birth defects has been noted in identical twins. While this may imply hereditary mechanisms, some surprising evidence from animal experiments suggests that identical twinning itself may be influenced by environmental factors.

In general, birth defects occur two to three times more often in twin than in single births. The United States Collaborative Perinatal Project — an intensive study of all births over a fixed period — obtained information on 1195 twins. Some 219, about 18 percent of them, had minor and major birth infirmities, with more than one defect present in a vast majority of these infants. It appeared, however, that this large figure was caused for the most part by identical rather than nonidentical twins. Also, birth defects occurred more frequently in black than in white twins, and more among male than female twins.

Both members of an identical pair are frequently subject to the same defects, suggesting, of course, a hereditary influence.

Heart defects, especially, fall into this category. In contrast, it is exceedingly rare to find both twins, either nonidentical or identical, affected by a severe brain and skull defect called anencephaly (see Chapters 9 and 16). This observation further suggests the important role of unknown environmental factors as the cause of this defect.

Understanding the occurrence of chromosomal defects in twins is even more difficult. Without going into a complicated explanation, suffice it to say that chromosomal defects may occur in both members of a pair, in either identical or nonidentical twins. One author studying the frequency of Down's syndrome in twins found that 159 sets had been reported. Of all these sets of twins, only one twin was affected in 155 of the sets, the remaining four having both twins affected with mongolism. Another chromosomal defect that affects males and is characterized by an extra X chromosome (Klinefelter's syndrome, see Chapter 2) is more likely to affect both members of a twin pair. Indeed, a higher frequency of twinning has been noted in the brothers and sisters of affected people with Klinefelter's syndrome.

Fused (Siamese) Twins

A morbid fascination will probably always attend the birth of twins joined together at some part of their bodies. They are called Siamese because of a pair of twins, Chang and Eng, born in Siam, joined at the hips, who later joined Barnum's circus in the United States. Such twins occur about once in 33,000 to 165,000 births and most commonly are joined together at the chest. All such joined twins have the same sex and almost invariably have associated birth defects. About 70 percent of them are female. (Curious and totally unexplained is the fact that twins in chickens are invariably female.) The most likely reason for Siamese twins is the incomplete separation of the dividing cells following fertilization of a single egg. Most now believe that unknown but definite environmental influences affect this incomplete fission. Certain drugs may cause the same phenomenon of conjoined twins in hamsters, and a diminished oxygen concentration or simply raised water temperatures may be the cause in zebra fish. There does not, however, appear to be any clear hereditary factor recognized thus far that would predispose an individual couple to have fused twins.

On occasion, during the development of joined twins, the lack of separation may be quite bizarre. Incredible freaks may now and then be born as "monsters" with two heads and one body, or one head and two bodies, or one body and four arms and four legs, and so forth. These "monsters" are not usually born alive, but if so, rarely live more than a few hours.

Death in Twins

An increased rate of death in twins at the time of birth or soon thereafter is well recognized and relates mainly to the higher rate of premature delivery. The occurrence of death in the first month of life is seven times higher for twins than for single births, and the likelihood of death while still in the womb is three times greater. It turns out that identical twins have a much greater risk of dying than nonidentical twins during the first month of life. As could be expected, most commonly the second delivered twin is at the greatest disadvantage in terms of survival and development. The use of instruments for delivery, the length of anesthesia, and the lack of oxygen associated with the delay all adversely affect the outcome for the second twin. Sometimes, in about 1 in 1000 deliveries, twins actually interlock during delivery; a complication that leads to death of both babies in about one-third of such cases.

Pregnancy with Twins

Family history aside, it is not really possible to predict who will have twins. It has been noticed, however, that on the average, women who weigh more in relation to their height *before* pregnancy are more apt to have twins than their slimmer peers.

A woman or her doctor is usually alerted to a twin pregnancy by the larger womb size, faster and bigger weight gain, and the actual discernment of multiple fetal parts during an abdominal examination.

Early diagnosis is important, though this is seldom accomplished. Mothers carrying twins need greater care. Twins who are heavier in the womb are diagnosed early, and weigh more when born, which is good. The smaller, late-diagnosed twins are more wont to be born prematurely, which is not good. Failure to diagnose twins at all before labor poses greater hazards to the second one delivered, for various reasons including harm caused by drugs used to contract the uterus after delivery.

CHAPTER 27

Should the Defective Newborn
Be Allowed to Die?

THE BABY was born with Down's syndrome (mongolism) at the Johns Hopkins Hospital in Baltimore. Within hours after birth it became apparent that some intestinal complication was present. The diagnosis of duodenal atresia (a birth defect causing complete obstruction at the exit of the stomach into the intestine) was made and the parents advised that operation was necessary for the correction of this obstruction. The parents elected not to have surgery on this child, who if operated upon would virtually certainly have survived albeit with moderate-severe mental retardation. The untreated baby slowly starved to death over a two-week period.

This experience, devastating for all concerned, took place in a highly renowned institution with the highest possible standard of care. Needless to say, this was not the first time that a baby was allowed to die in a newborn nursery or intensive care unit. Doctors at yet another distinguished institution, the Yale–New Haven Hospital in Connecticut, reported in the *New England Journal of Medicine*, in 1973, that 43 (14 percent) of 299 infants admitted to the newborn intensive care unit in one year with irreparable damage or defects were allowed to die. In newborn intensive care nurseries the world over, I have seen the tragic situations those doctors faced: babies with open spine defects who would never be able to walk or have bladder and bowel control; with severe hydrocephalus who would be severely mentally retarded and blind; babies who through brain damage from lack of oxygen, hemorrhage, or other causes would have been spastic, totally paralyzed or unable even to turn over in bed; or babies with severe genetic defects that heralded, without a doubt, profound mental retardation and vegetative existence as well as pain and suffering.

Just a few years ago, parents, doctors, and society did not have to confront the situations we face so often today, where advances in medical technology enable the genetically or otherwise defective child to be kept alive either with a respirator or by other artificial means. The difficulties are compounded further because while in certain cases it is possible to be absolutely sure of a disastrous outcome, in others a degree of uncertainty in the prognosis cannot be denied.

The Present Posture of the Law

In the United States and elsewhere, laws are designed for the protection of human life and clearly extend to defective newborns as well as young or old adults. The legal constraints on medical procedure are backed up with threats of punishment for noncompliance. Hence, it is clear that all participants caught in the dilemma of trying to decide the fate of a defective newborn place themselves in danger. Parents, doctors, nurses, hospital administrators, and various other members of the hospital staff, despite their good intentions, may be liable for crimes that range from murder to manslaughter, including child abuse, neglect, or even conspiracy to withhold medical care leading to injury or death of the newborn. Burdened by such liabilities, we cannot cease to admire the courage and motivations of those entrusted with and dedicated to the care of the seriously ill newborn. So explicit is the law that even advising or recommending to parents may expose the physician to legal suit on the basis of conspiracy to commit homicide, for example, by withholding treatment. While no parent or doctor, to my knowledge, has been successfully prosecuted for withholding care from a defective newborn, that is no comfort for those taking chances. There certainly have been prosecutions for the active killing of defective offspring.

Torture for the Parents

Armchair critics abound in this as well as in other painful controversies. Consider yourself, however, as the parent of a newborn infant with grave defects that will allow the child only a vegetative existence in the future. What would your reactions be? The doctor caring for the infant, by law, would have to inform you and your spouse that you may be criminally liable for making a nontreatment decision; that even if you do not wish to keep the child, you are obliged to in the face of the law until at least formal alternative arrangements have been worked out where possible. Even if you and your spouse decide to take the risk of prosecution, the doctor is legally obliged to take steps aimed at saving the child. He might simply have to report the case to the child welfare officer or follow the child abuse law reporting scheme, or the hospital itself might have to initiate neglect proceedings. The parents find themselves more entrapped when they realize that even by discharging the doctor from the case they do not avoid criminal liability, because by submitting to their wishes or with knowledge of their intentions, the doctors again are forced to communicate with the authorities.

Why then have there not been prosecutions of either doctors or parents in these tragic situations when clearly it is totally illegal to decide to withhold treatment of a gravely defective newborn? The answer lies, thankfully, in the small number of parents, doctors, or nurses who pressure the public prosecutor and, moreover, in the wisdom and humanity of prosecutors who ignore the situations. The Edelin trial, however, involving an obstetrician accused of manslaughter of a fetus during a routine abortion, may signal an end to studied prosecutorial indifference. Any such change would be an extremely sad eventuality for all parents having gravely defective offspring.

Unfortunately, in the eyes of many people there are simply no grounds for withholding treatment; but these are probably mostly individuals who have never had to face personally these soul-destroying decisions.

The Defective Child

Consideration should first be given to the defective infant. He or she may survive, tortured by endless weeks, months, or years by all manner of tubes, needles, catheters, and so on, as well as by the associated pain, suffering, and indignity. The question may justifiably be asked if that child or any of us ourselves would demand the continuation of artificial life-support systems? While the child has a right to life, the courts have already indicated that that right extends to life with a normal and healthy mind and body. Ascribing the responsibilities of such events to a higher being does not release you or the doctors or nurses from the grave difficulties encountered in caring for such defective infants. Indeed, the Roman Catholic Church accepts that judgment may be employed when *extraordinary* measures are required to preserve and extend life. Most Protestant and Jewish theologians would concur with this view, drawing attention, however, to the difficulty in distinguishing between ordinary and extraordinary measures.

The Family

Consideration of the family and any other living siblings of the defective infant is crucial. I have discussed, in detail, the consequences to a family faced with a seriously defective or mentally retarded child (see Chapter 1). A recent study of families of children with open spine defects showed that 62 percent were judged to have made poor adjustments, and that 43 percent of the parents were divorced or separated. And of course there is no measure of the sadness and emotional chaos. However, other studies on similarly affected families found fewer cases of broken marriages and indications that many families were willing to make great efforts and sacrifices for the defective child's sake.

Certainly it can be argued that families may give up their obligations to care for a defective child. Odious as that possibility would appear to be, it might for some be less traumatic than the contemplation of withholding vital treatment. It would seem that consideration of the siblings is frequently less compelling than concern for the welfare of the defective child.

In such situations, the physician represents more than just

"an interested party." Personal feelings aside — and considerable self-discipline is required — the physician knows what lies in store for the parents and the defective child. Cognizant of the likely future and concerned about the general health and welfare of the family, the physician will realize the degree of devastation in store for both the defective child and the family. Although predisposed to the idea of death with dignity, and to avoidance of the torture to all concerned, the doctor finds himself prevented by law from following a parent's wishes that he abandon extraordinary or heroic measures to save the life of the defective child.

Many elements go into the physician's decision. Professor I. David Todres and his colleagues at the Massachusetts General Hospital evaluated some of the pediatricians' attitudes to surgery on infants with Down's syndrome or open spine defects. In their questionnaire-study, they showed that if the baby had Down's syndrome and duodenal atresia, 50.7 percent of pediatricians did *not* advocate surgery. Of those advocating surgery, Catholics were in the majority. Almost 20 percent of those advocating surgery indicated that they would try to get a court order. The general conclusions of the study were that the physician's attitude in advocating or withholding surgery depended on his or her religious persuasion and activity and on his or her age and degree of specialization.

The State

Society, too, has a vested interest in decisions concerning the disposition of the defective newborn. There is a general empathy felt for all individuals who are subjected to pain and suffering. Hence, society could make available facilities for the care of the gravely defective child and ultimately for the institutionalization that so often follows. Resources for long-term care, however, are scarce the world over; objectively speaking, certain other health priorities have to be recognized. Moreover, institutions for the severely deformed or defective are in poor repute in some countries. When it is realized that the projected cost of lifetime institutional care for one child born with Down's syndrome will exceed $250,000, the argument is advanced that instead of spending literally billions of dollars for the care of seriously defective offspring, those financial resources should be put to better use, such as the prevention of such defects. Sadly enough, if such a priority should take over, many others, like the elderly or the chronically sick, may get hurt in the process. Hence, the state becomes inexorably involved in making comparative assessments as it tries not to deviate from its fundamental commitment to the safety and sanctity of all persons.

Decisions and Decisions: Who Shall Die? The Four Alternatives

1. The Present System

Professor Robert Burt of the University of Michigan Law School has argued eloquently that the current system of formal legality remain. That is to say, doctors, parents, nurses, and everyone involved in the care of the defective newborn should continue to operate under the threat of prosecution for withholding treatment from any defective newborn, laboring on in the shadow of possible and only occasional court action. He has indicated that from his perspective this is probably "the best choice among bad choices."

2. The Death Committee

Consider yourself, for a moment, as the parent of a gravely defective newborn faced with the decision that would allow the surgeon to operate or the physician to withhold crucial treatment. Could you imagine yourself either appearing before or submitting in writing your views to a committee? Such a committee, made up no doubt of laymen, physicians, theologians, and nurses, would be charged with the responsibility as an impartial body of making decisions regarding the withholding of treatment for gravely defective newborns. No such action would be permissible without their concurrence with the decision of the parents and attending doctor.

The difficulties of establishing such a committee, developing its procedural matters, having it available in the middle of the night and at other frequent and unusual hours, could pose serious dilemmas. Setting up such a committee as the decision maker might be regarded by many as an untenable infringement on their rights and their own wisdom. Nevertheless, in the decision handed down by the Supreme Court of New Jersey in the Karen Quinlan case, just such an ethics committee was discussed.

One other approach is to appoint an advocate who would represent the interests of the child in discussions between the parents and the doctor. This system would be clearly more satisfactory than the death committee approach, but would suffer in one basic way. The relationship of the parents to their doctor, based on confidentiality and trust, could be impaired. But many maintain that the parents are too emotionally involved to make objective assessments and decisions, that the physician is insufficiently equipped for profound ethical evaluations, and that without the third party advocate, the interests of the child would not be adequately represented.

3. The State as Decision Maker

The state acting through the courts and legislatures could easily make mandatory an official application process through state-appointed bodies empowered to consider and to enforce decisions relating to life or death. Could you picture yourself, as a parent of a defective newborn, applying for consideration to this euthanasia committee? The objections are the same as delineated above for the death committee. This time, however, there is an even graver implication in that the state would then become implicated in the relative assessment of worthiness to live! The state might decide, in a not unusual approach, to establish a certain classification of diseases for nontreatment. One danger of such an approach is the enormous variation in genetic disease. For example, a child with spina bifida (open-spine) may have a defect that is totally correctable by surgery, enabling normal control of bowel and bladder as well as walking. Other cases with the same diagnosis, however, can differ after surgery, from total paraplegia and no bowel or bladder control to many variations of partial cure.

An even greater danger of having state control over such decisions is the implicit hazard to our political principles: if the state should suddenly be empowered to decide who shall live and who shall die, we would then have moved from a democracy to a dictatorship. Heaven knows how such a policy might be extended to include eventually living handicapped individuals, institutionalized persons, people with mental disorders, various types of criminals, the elderly, the sick, certain religious sects, and finally, people of different ethnic origins!

4. Parents and Doctor as Decision Makers

No one is more concerned than the parents of a newborn baby about its welfare. Parents are indeed recognized in law as having enormous powers over the welfare of their offspring, and it would make more sense that this parental authority remain unchallenged. Their relationship with their child's doctor, based on confidentiality and trust, provides a solid basis for the resolution of sensitive and difficult problems. Parents and doctors working together with the best interests of the child at heart are undoubtedly best equipped to make these extremely trying decisions. You will recall that the decisions to be made are those of omission and not commission; this means that the parents and the doctor decide to *withhold* treatment of a particular nature, as opposed to specifically administering a drug or poison to kill the child. Some would argue that there is no philosophical difference, no action can be construed as action, and it can, therefore, be considered as killing the child.

As we have said earlier, one important difficulty is the emotional shock and distress enveloping parents at such moments, and the differing attitudes of physicians to life and death — their own varying personal beliefs, experience generally with children with severe disabilities, religious affiliations, and so forth.

I believe that parents and physicians *acting together* should be allowed broader discretion in their decision making concerning the treatment or nontreatment of defective newborns. For them to have to do this under the threat of criminal prosecution is untenable.

Conclusion

The pain and suffering of a newborn with grave birth defects, the devastation caused in the family, and the implications for society as a whole call for a definite policy in regard to decision making, and one that is legally safe. Of the four alternatives presented, it is clear that the present situation, with parents and doctors under continual threat of prosecution, is most unsatisfactory. The third party technique or death committee is no better than giving the government the power of arbitrary euthanasia. It would seem best for parents and doctors to determine, case by case, what should be done or not done. They are best situated to evaluate the suffering of the child and to allow the child to die with dignity in the most humane way. I believe, together with doctors at the Yale–New Haven Hospital and elsewhere, that such decisions should be made independent of the law. I am in agreement with those who feel that if selection for nontreatment is in violation of the law, then the law should be changed.

CHAPTER 28

Test-Tube Babies — A Reality?

AN OBSTETRICIAN IN LEEDS, ENGLAND, announced, in 1974, that he was aware of three healthy children who had each been born after fertilization of an ovum by sperm in a test tube, the fertilized egg then being implanted into the mother's womb. He was insistent in refusing to divulge any more details, maintaining that his duty was to protect the privacy of the parents and offspring involved. Hence, the validity of this claim remains in question. Nevertheless, because of technological developments in the understanding of control of reproduction, it is clear that the whole process is perfectly feasible and may indeed have already occurred successfully.

Why, you might ask, is it necessary to go the route of fertilizing human eggs in a test tube?

Who Would Benefit?

We already noted, in Chapter 13, that some 10 to 12 percent of married couples are infertile. Most causes of infertility can be traced to defects in the woman's reproductive system. A significant number of those women whose gynecological problems are responsible for infertility have blocked Fallopian tubes. These connect a woman's ovaries with the uterus, and the ovum passes through them on its way to fertilization and possible implantation in the womb. One conservative estimate counts over 20,000 women in the United Kingdom with blocked tubes, and at least seven times as many in the United States. Moreover, the number is increasing because of the current epidemic proportions of venereal disease, especially gonorrhea, in the United States and elsewhere.

Women with blocked Fallopian tubes have, of course, normal ovaries containing normal eggs. Hence, if it were possible to circumvent the blocked tubes and transfer an ovum from the ovary into the uterus, where it could be fertilized, the problem would be solved. However, no artificial tubes have yet been successfully transplanted. An alternative has hence been developed: the removal of an ovum from the ovary and its fertilization in a test tube by the husband's own sperm. After a few days, this fertilized ovum is transferred to the mother's womb, which has especially been prepared for it by the prospective mother taking hormones by mouth.

Besides the benefit to infertile couples, the research backing this technique may bring us more profound understanding of human genetic disorders and possibly even the development of new methods of contraception. It has been emphasized that women having babies conceived in a "test tube" from their own husband's sperm are able to have their *own* children, in contradistinction to artificial insemination by donor.

There are also some women — and the number is very small — who are unable to have babies because they do not produce ova at all. In such cases, it would be necessary to obtain ova from a donor. The donated ovum would then be placed in a test tube and fertilized by the husband's sperm.

The State of the Art

Rabbits were used, as long ago as 1890, in experiments for transferring ova. Since that time, successful transfers have been made in at least seven warm-blooded animals including pigs, mice, hamsters, and various farm animals. Initially, the fertilized ovum was placed into the womb of the recipient female animal by an operation. A high rate (up to 90 percent) of successful transfer of fertilized ova was achieved with this technique. But, later, the less traumatic technique of proceeding through the female genital tract was studied. Successful transfers of fertilized ova through the genital tract and the cervix of cattle have been achieved in at least 50 percent of attempts. Similar success has been achieved with this approach in mice. Early research already indicates that it can also be successful in human beings.

It is extremely important that after the birth of many hundreds of offspring in different animal species, no *induced* congenital defects attributable to manipulation of ova and sperm have been found. Nor is there indication of any increase in the frequency of birth defects.

As far as the human female is concerned, if transfer of a fertilized ovum has not already been successfully achieved, resulting in a normally developing fetus and normal delivery, then such an eventuality must be imminent. The general techniques and approaches appear to have been largely resolved. Various hormones are first given to the woman in order to control the growth and development of the ovum and the process leading to release of the ovum, or ovulation. Just before the female is expected to ovulate, a tiny telescopic instrument, called a laparoscope, is inserted through the abdominal wall. Through this instrument, it is possible to collect the ovum directly from the ovary. It can then be fertilized in a tube by sperm collected from the husband, developed in special nutrient fluids for a few days, then transferred through the vagina and cervix into the hormonally prepared uterus. The mother would continue to take hormones to support the early stages of fetal development. Thus far, success in obtaining human ova from the ovaries via the laparoscope has been better than 50 percent.

Ethical and Legal Dilemmas

Not unexpectedly much debate has centered around laboratory fertilization of the female ovum. Medically, it is called in vitro fertilization and is abbreviated as IVF. Theologians and others concerned with ethics have questioned the morality of procreation in a test tube. Calling such technology absolutely immoral, some have even maintained that it could erode the very basis of marriage and even pose a threat to society. The argument has even been advanced that since infertility is not a disease, IVF aims to satisfy *desires* instead of treating *illnesses* and therefore cannot be morally condoned. Yet some well-known ethicists considering the balance of benefit versus possible harm have concluded that the innate need and constitutional right of women to bear children fully justifies the use of IVF.

Should Government Be Involved?

The state could certainly make the conception of babies in a test tube illegal, under the guise of protecting individuals from harm caused by others, by maintaining that society has a right to protect individuals from self-inflicted damage or even from exposure to immoral practices. Such laws would be extremely difficult to enforce, would not be justifiable, and, indeed, would probably affront the duly constituted rights of women. The courts have repeatedly acted in recent years to ensure that the decisions of couples to conceive and have babies remain a private matter and not under the jurisdiction of the court. In this context, conceiving babies in a test tube would appear to be a matter of privacy and confidentiality between the parents and physician.

State involvement in some defined areas of IVF, however, would be not only acceptable but desirable. If we assume there will be continued progress with IVF, then it will behoove the state to ensure the highest standards of safety in its laboratory aspects. For example, it is likely that eventually ova banks would be established in which human ova could be stored frozen for many years. There already are sperm banks. Parenthetically, you could imagine the day when women place in storage a supply of ova, after which they have their tubes tied. A new approach to contraception would then have arrived! Moreover, women would then be in a position to dictate to the very day when they wish an ovum to be fertilized — the ultimate in family planning!

The Married Couple

The married couple are unlikely to cause legal problems, unless things go wrong, such as surgical complications during efforts to obtain the ovum from the ovary. Or, because of laboratory error, the wrong sperm could be utilized in fertilization. Or, finally, the couple could claim that they were not fully informed if they discovered that the baby had a major birth defect.

The Physician and the Laboratory Staff

While operating in good faith, the physician may still be sued for alleged negligence during surgical maneuvers or for alleged mishandling of either the ovum or sperm when obtained. Due care would have to be exercised by the physician to obtain both written and verbal informed consent from the couple. Nevertheless, all complications can never be foreseen and such documents may be of limited value. Certainly the technology would have to have been sufficiently advanced as to prevent any action on the basis of human experimentation by the doctor.

The Fertilized Ovum

All experimental evidence currently points away from the probability of damage to ova in the process. Nevertheless, it could happen. The rights of the fertilized ovum are not likely to be operative until the period of viability has been reached, about 24 to 28 weeks of pregnancy. In some jurisdictions a baby would have to be delivered alive before any action could be pursued. Clearly, the fetus would have the rights that apply to the period of viability recognized by the particular jurisdiction. Hence, the fetus could inherit and has been seen to have state rights (see detailed discussion in Chapter 17). Moreover, the advocate for the child could sue the doctor if the child was born with some birth defect, if some activity by the physician could be brought into question. Incredibly, the advocate could even sue the couple! Such a situation could develop if, for example, the mother had failed to obtain immunization against German measles, was exposed during pregnancy, and the child was born with serious defects.

German measles or other known causes aside, the child conceived in a test tube might be born with a birth defect, though it would be extremely difficult to prove the cause in most such cases.

The Third Party Donor

Inevitably, there will be a number of women who are unable to provide their own ovum, and it will be necessary to obtain ova from donors. Such women, just like blood donors, might insist on a fee. All the other legal paraphernalia concerning privacy, confidentiality, and other aspects discussed for artificial insemination (see Chapter 13) would apply equally in this situation. The ovum donor, for example, would not be allowed to know the identity of the married couple or of the child born subsequently.

Justified genetic reasons for donation of ova from third parties would be respected. For example, a woman who is a known carrier of a sex-linked disorder, such as muscular dystrophy, might not wish to pass on the disease or face abortion. She might, therefore, elect to have a third party donate an ovum, which she could carry in her own womb. It is just conceivable that ultimately, as lawyer Philip Reilly of the University of Yale Law School has suggested, ova from women of superior intelligence could be selected for the intention of having children with superior intellects.

The Third Party Recipient

Sometimes a woman has normal ovaries but is unable to have a pregnancy because of a birth defect of her womb, its removal because of a tumor or for other reasons, or her inability to retain a pregnancy. In such cases, the couple might choose to have the wife's ovum removed from her ovary and fertilized in the laboratory by her husband's sperm. The fertilized ovum would then be implanted in another woman who had volunteered to carry this couple's offspring through pregnancy. "Wombs for rent" is only one of the likely developments in this process that truly bristles with complexities.

Even though there would be a legal contract between the married couple and the recipient woman, a number of problems could turn up. The pregnancy could go badly for the surrogate mother, who could then decided to abort the pregnancy on the grounds of her concern for her personal health. Could she be sued for breach of contract for not carrying the other couple's offspring to term? If the child were born defective, could she be sued for not exercising due care? Could there be contractual clauses forcing certain restrictions on the surrogate mother during pregnancy? If she kept the baby after birth, could she be arrested for kidnaping? Under whose name would the child be registered at birth in the face of the law? Would such a child have the constitutional right to know his or her origin? (In Scotland, for example, adopted children, by law, are able to trace their origins and their biological parents.)

Just in case you think all these ideas are quite fanciful, there is at least one instance in Texas where an inquiry has already arisen from a couple who wish to have a child with their own genes, but carried by a surrogate mother because the real mother has had a partial hysterectomy and is unable to carry any pregnancy. Fees have even been discussed, and there are some that believe that $10,000 to $15,000 is a reasonable premium.

The whole discussion about test-tube babies and IVF serves to remind us that science moves much faster than law. This disparity in momentum is within the very nature of both disciplines, making it extremely difficult to anticipate major scientific advances and to formulate the necessary legal guidelines that would diminish the chance of someone getting hurt.

CHAPTER 29

The Future

IT GOES WITHOUT SAYING that medical genetic research is the
key to the understanding and possible cure of many diseases.
Cancer, heart disease, allergic disorders, hypertension, many
birth defects, and inborn errors of body chemistry, to name
but a few, are critical areas for likely progress. Only through
increasing government and private foundation support for research in genetics will it be possible to ensure this progress,
and to apply the information gathered for the benefit of both
individual and public health.

Genetic Engineering: Donating or Removing Genes

It would be a phenomenal breakthrough if it became possible
to isolate human genes. Such isolated genes could then be
donated specifically to individuals with a particular gene that
was defective. Theoretically, this could be achieved by excis-
ing the defective gene from the affected individual and replacing it with a normal one. Actually, to synthesize genes, to
excise them, and then replace them would be the ultimate in
genetic engineering. And we are now not talking science
fiction.

It is already possible to inject donor cells into a mouse embryo. These cells multiply and are later found in different organs in the mouse. It has also been shown in animals that
chromosomes or an entire cell nucleus can be removed from
an ovum and replaced by a nucleus from a donor. The offspring in such a situation would display characteristics of the
donor. These approaches provide a way actually to *cure* genetic disease by active intervention even before the potential
person is more than a few cells old!

One slightly different effort at gene therapy was made in West Germany in recent years. It had been noted that a certain virus infection, incidentally found in laboratory workers, induced a high level of a certain enzyme. When two sisters with a rare biochemical hereditary disorder were found deficient in this particular enzyme, the physicians decided, in the face of no known treatment, to infect both girls with the particular virus. The idea was simply to have the virus create the missing enzyme, thereby "curing" the disease in both girls. This experiment failed by making no detectable difference. Moreover, it generated a tremendous controversy because the physicians had failed to establish the safety and advisability of the technique, some even suggesting that infecting the girls with the virus could ultimately cause tumors.

Such experiments based on technical advances have unfortunately raised serious questions about the safety with which they can be pursued, since the technology would be developed by using bacteria and viruses. The implicit danger is that by tinkering with the basic genetic apparatus of the human being, new diseases will be spawned, which could create a major health hazard, and that dramatic scientific breakthroughs can open up a Pandora's box of situations. Abuses of new discoveries could be disastrous for whole nations. Politically, the implication is that by manipulating the genes, an awesome power may be placed in the hands of a few who, it is said, could effectively threaten mankind.

In this connection, specific guidelines have been issued by the United States government that will govern the conduct of government-supported research on what is called recombinant DNA molecules, which are molecules resulting from the recombination in cell-free systems of segments of DNA or genes.

Scientists the world over have not been blind to the potential dangers of such research, and have cooperated with governments in developing guidelines such as those referred to above. Public concern and anxiety have, however, not been mollified. In Cambridge, Massachusetts, scientists at Harvard University have found themselves assailed by the city council who, on behalf of the city, has been concerned about the safety of the community in which such research is pursued. One would hope that the procedures and safety guidelines to be used will reassure this and other communities. The potential benefits of this work in molecular biology cannot, and should not, be underestimated.

These ongoing and planned studies are aimed at learning about the structure and function of genes. The work may involve artificially joining genes from one species to another, for example, humans and bacteria. The new molecules so formed could then be inserted into bacteria for mass production. This might make it possible to "manufacture" insulin, human growth hormone, and other valuable substances inexpensively.

Mapping the Genes

Knowing which gene to excise and replace would depend upon knowing its exact location on a particular chromosome. Various ingenious techniques have been devised to determine the location of specific genes on chromosomes. One continuing fruitful approach is the fusing of human and animal (e.g., mouse, hamster or rat) cells. Impressive progress has been made. For example, the gene for the enzyme that when deficient causes Tay-Sachs disease is located on chromosome #15. Other gene locations include chromosome #1 for the Rh blood group, chromosome #9 for ABO blood groups, and chromosome #19 for a gene that may make you susceptible, if not immunized, to poliomyelitis. There are, perhaps, some two and a half million genes, the location of only a handful being known thus far. You may anticipate enormous progress in gene mapping in the future.

Cloning

A clone (or group of cells) originates from a single cell. The process is easily achieved by growing cells in the laboratory. Science fiction writers first generated the idea that since each cell in the body has a complete genetic code or blueprint for life, simply inducing a single cell to divide in a continuous process would eventually lead to the full development of a new individual; moreover, the new individual would be an exact copy of the person whose cell was used — and all this without the help of the opposite sex!

It would be safe to say that simply *growing humans* from their own donated single cells will remain a science fiction idea for the foreseeable future.

Genetics, Society, and the Future

Given the continuation and increase of the critically important government funding for genetic research, tremendous advances can be anticipated. The distant goals include, of course, complete eradication of the disease to which we are so frequently genetically predisposed.

Progress in the prenatal diagnosis of genetic disease must be allowed to continue, making more and more diseases identifiable. Treatment of the fetus via the mother or directly in the womb may diminish the need for abortion. Serious constraints, such as the prevention of studies on the fetus to be aborted, now exist in some states in the United States. The ultimate victims of such laws are the defective children who suffer, the anguished parents, and the taxpayers who pay the institutional bills.

Within a decade or two, it is likely that amniocentesis, already shown to be a safe procedure, will be available to every pregnant woman desirous of excluding diagnosable birth defects. The approach (which as I stated earlier I would not permit in my laboratories) of fetal sex determination and abortion solely on a family planning whim will undoubtedly be replaced by techniques that allow sex selection *prior* to conception.

Ultimately each of us might carry a gene identity card. Blood tests during childhood might be used to determine which hereditary diseases we carry, which we may be predisposed to, as well as other usual information regarding future childbearing. I hope that long before any of this happens state governments will provide young couples planning to

marry with a pamphlet indicating the need for genetic counseling *prior* to marriage. While I failed to secure even this
arrangement in Boston (because of the fear that couples might
choose abortion as an option after genetic counseling), I hope
others will succeed.

Certainly you should have the freedom to know if you are at
risk for having a child with birth defects or mental retardation, and not be stifled by segments of society that interfere
with your choice among all the options. Moreover, I hope
that society will never dictate to you that personal choice, but
rather respect your own religious or other scruples — even if
your decision is to have defective children!

My commitment in writing this book is a testament to my
conviction that access to knowledge and the freedom to use it
should be unassailable. Only if you are fully informed, only if
you *know your genes* will you be able to make constructive,
rational decisions that will benefit your children and their
descendants. In the context of shaping the destinies of the yet-
to-be-born, the words of President John F. Kennedy apply with
a special force:

The future belongs to those who prepare for it.

Questions You Thought
of Asking

INNUMERABLE QUESTIONS must have crossed your mind while reading this book. The purpose of this text was not to provide an encyclopedic coverage of genetic disease nor to masquerade as a genetic textbook or an introduction to biology. Its fundamental themes were to alert you to the importance of genetic disease as it affects you and your family and to provide insights into what steps you might take to foreclose the likelihood of personal tragedies. This section is devoted to answering questions you might like to have asked and that have, in fact, been asked of me repeatedly over the years.

A few people in our family have allergy problems such as eczema and asthma. How important are the hereditary aspects in allergy?

The predisposition or tendency to become allergic is inherited rather than the specific allergy itself. How this is exactly effected is unknown, except that the body's immune system (which makes antibodies) is probably involved. Studies from the Swedish Twin Registry of 7000 like-sexed pairs of twins over forty years of age and 2400 identical twins showed that both members of an identical twin pair had allergy in 20 to 25 percent of the time. This figure suggests a lesser influence of genetic control than suggested by previous family studies. The best figures available show the following risks for children becoming allergic when one or both parents are already allergic:

	Both Parents Allergic (%)	One Parent Allergic (%)	Neither Parent Allergic (%)
Risks of child becoming allergic	75	50	
(from 3 different studies)	60	40	} 10 to 20
	40	30	

The allergy may vary from simple eczema, to asthma, to allergic reactions to drugs or foods, and so on. One parent, for example, may be allergic to a drug, while the child may take that drug with impunity, but be severely allergic to cats or dogs, and so on.

My father and my maternal grandmother both had emphysema. Am I at risk for developing emphysema as well?

Many people who develop emphysema do so following chronic bronchitis, usually caused by asthma or cigarette smoking. Individuals predisposed to asthma and bronchitis may be that way because of a genetic predisposition. There is no way at present, however, to provide any sensible guidance about the risk of emphysema to you in the face of some kind of family history.

There is, however, a condition characterized by a specific deficiency of a protein called alpha$_1$-antitrypsin. This deficiency is definitely transmitted as a hereditary trait. Those individuals who have deficient alpha$_1$-antitrypsin activity in their body fluids have a high risk of developing chronic obstructive lung disease (emphysema), usually starting during the fourth decade of life. To give you at least some idea of how complicated the matter is, some 23 different subtypes of this disorder have been recognized. An individual with one of these particular subtypes may carry a high risk (50 percent) of developing chronic obstructive lung disease. Cigarette smoking in these particular individuals may accelerate the deterioration of lung function. It is interesting that babies born with this genetic subtype have a 20 to 30 percent risk of developing hepatitis in the newborn period and subsequent cirrhosis of the liver. Deficiency of alpha$_1$-antitrypsin is not rare. One large population study estimated that this deficiency may be present in 3 to 6 percent of the population.

Is baldness inherited?

There is no doubt that certain types of baldness are inherited. Pattern baldness is perhaps the best example and is expressed as a thinning of the hair at the temples and, when severe, is also associated with baldness at the top of the head with hair remaining on the sides. This type of baldness is found almost exclusively in males, and appears to be passed from father to son but usually not to daughters. The pattern of inheritance is probably dominant and, as such, really limited to males. Some sons of bald fathers, however, do not become bald, as you might perhaps expect.

Is the Sudden Infant Death Syndrome (SIDS) hereditary?

Also called crib death, the SIDS is a disorder in which apparently healthy babies are found dead in their cribs without any warning or prior illness. SIDS is probably the most common single cause of death in babies between one week and one year of age in the United States; approximately 10,000 apparently well babies die each year from this cause. Thus far, innumerable theories have been proposed, but the real cause and mechanisms responsible for SIDS have not been recognized. In late 1975, a team working at the National Heart and Lung Institute, Bethesda, Maryland, reported that an abnormality in the electrocardiogram was present in at least 1 member of 11 (26 percent) sets of parents out of the 42 sets they had studied, each of whom had had at least one infant with SIDS. Moreover, they observed a similar abnormality in the electrocardiograms in 39 percent of the siblings of infants who had died with SIDS. These observations strongly suggest that at least for some kinds of SIDS cases the existence of a dominant hereditary factor (see Chapter 5) may be important, though it is extremely likely that a number of other different causes will also be found to explain SIDS. Much more research is still required to assess the genetic factors. Meanwhile, if you have tragically lost a child from crib death, it would seem reasonable to have electrocardiograms for yourself and your spouse.

Is handedness genetically transmitted?

It has been recognized for a long time that two right-handed parents have the least number of left-handed offspring, that two left-handed parents have the most left-handed offspring, and that couples, one of whom is left-handed, the other right-handed, have an intermediate number of children who are left-handed. These observations have clearly pointed to obvious parental influences on the development of handedness. Factors that mitigate against the parental influence being via genes is that the proportions of handedness in identical twins, nonidentical twins, and in brothers and sisters are roughly the same, following completely chance expectations. Currently, it seems most likely that parental environmental influence in child rearing is strongest in influencing the development of handedness. It may be significant that the frequency of left-handed children is higher when the mother is left-handed and the father right-handed than the other way around.

Could we predict the hair color of our next child?

The inheritance of hair color is complex. Dark-colored hair tends to dominate over lighter colored hair. Hence, it is likely that most children born of one parent with dark hair and one with light hair are most likely to have dark hair. The gene for red hair color operates separately from the gene for dark hair color and is generally recessive in nature. Hence, in general, you might expect all the children of red-headed parents to have red hair color. If, however, one of the red-headed parents is also carrying the gene for dark hair color, a variety of hair colors may eventuate in the offspring. If a black-haired individual marries a redhead, you might theoretically expect no red-headed offspring. However, if the black-haired individual carried the recessive gene for red hair, then half the children might be expected to be red-headed. It should be obvious that it is extremely difficult to predict hair color.

My husband and I have blue eyes. Will all our children have blue eyes?

The response is similar to that just given for hair color. In general, the genes for the darker colors tend to dominate over those for the lighter, but a whole range of shades and possibilities invariably exist, and predictions are generally not possible.

Can epilepsy be inherited?

There are innumerable causes of epilepsy varying from brain damage occurring to the fetus while in the womb, during delivery, or during life. A variety of different genetic disorders have epilepsy as their sole or major feature. Hence, no straightforward answer can be given to this question without carefully evaluating the family history, examinations, and special tests on the affected individual.

Both my parents are very overweight. Will I also be obese?

Body weight is undoubtedly determined by an interaction of genetic, environmental, and hormonal factors, which affect not only the size of fat cells, but also their number. There is evidence that certain ethnic groups have genes for obesity or for leanness. For example, the Papago Indians of southern Arizona, some Polynesian populations, and many Central and South American Indian tribes seem to possess a high frequency of genes for obesity. In contrast, certain tribes in Africa, such as the Watusi, have shown a higher tendency toward leanness.

Nevertheless, there are so many factors that influence body weight that to distinguish a particular genetic factor of consequence is extremely difficult. Certainly, nutritional, biochemical, genetic, psychological, social, and environmental factors have been clearly recognized in their relationship to the development of obesity. Among the most important of these may be how much is fed (and when) to the infant in the first weeks and months of life.

Notwithstanding recognition of the multiple causes of obesity, some evidence is available on those individuals who are overweight simply on the basis of overeating. (This is, in fact, true for almost all of us.) In addition, if one parent was obese, then it appears that there is a 40 to 50 percent chance of the children developing obesity. The likelihood rises to 70 to 80 percent if both parents were obese. These figures are in contrast to the only 8 to 9 percent of children who have parents of normal weight and are nevertheless obese. As expected, identical twins reared in the same environment show less difference in weight than do nonidentical twins. Interestingly, the weights of adopted children have shown no relationship to their foster parents, even though the children were adopted soon after birth.

Biochemical Diseases That Can Be Diagnosed Prenatally

Lipidoses

Cholesterol ester storage
  disease †
Fabry's disease *
Farber's disease †
Gaucher's disease *
Generalized gangliosidosis
  (GM₁ gangliosidosis type 1) *
Juvenile GM₁ gangliosidosis
  (GM₁ gangliosidosis type 2) *
Tay-Sachs disease
  (GM₂ gangliosidosis type 1) *
Sandhoff's disease
  (GM₂ gangliosidosis type 2) *

Juvenile GM₂ gangliosidosis
  (GM₂ gangliosidosis type 3) †
GM₃ sphingolipidystrophy †
Krabbe's disease (globoid cell
  leukodystrophy) *
Metachromatic leukodystrophy *
Niemann-Pick disease type A *
Niemann-Pick disease type B †
Niemann-Pick disease type C †
Refsum's disease †
Wolman's disease *

Mucopolysaccharidoses

MPS I — Hurler's syndrome*
MPS I — Scheie's syndrome †
MPS — Hurler/Scheie syndrome †
MPS II A — Hunter's syndrome *
MPS II B — Hunter's syndrome †
MPS III — Sanfilippo A syndrome *
  Sanfilippo B syndrome †

MPS IV — Morquio's syndrome †
MPS VI A — Maroteaux-Lamy
  syndrome †
MPS VII — β-glucuronidase
  deficiency †

Amino Acid and Related Disorders

Argininosuccinic aciduria *
Aspartylglucosaminuria †
Citrullinemia †
Congenital hyperammonemia †
Cystathionine synthase deficiency
  (homocystinuria) †
Cystathioninuria †
Cystinuria *
Hartnup disease †

Histidinemia †
Hypervalinemia †
Iminoglycinuria †
Isoleucine catabolism
  disorder †
Isovaleric acidemia †
Maple syrup urine disease
  Severe infantile *
  Intermittent †

* prenatal diagnosis possible
† prenatal diagnosis potentially possible

Methylmalonic aciduria
  Unresponsive to vitamin B_{12} †
  Responsive to vitamin B_{12} *
Methylenetetrahydrofolate reductase
  deficiency †
Ornithine-α-ketoacid transaminase
  deficiency †
Propionyl-CoA-carboxylase
  deficiency (ketotic
  hyperglycinemia) †

Succinyl-CoA: 3-ketoacid-CoA-
  transferase deficiency †
Vitamin B_{12} metabolic defect †

Disorders of Carbohydrate Metabolism

Fucosidosis †
Galactokinase deficiency †
Galactosemia *
Glucose-6-phoshate dehydrogenase
  deficiency †
Glycogen storage disease
  (type II) †

Glycogen storage disease (type III) †
Glycogen storage disease (type IV) *
Mannosidosis †
Phosphohexose isomerase
  deficiency †
Pyruvate decarboxylase deficiency †
Pyruvate dehydrogenase deficiency †

Miscellaneous Hereditary Disorders

Acatalasemia †
Acute intermittent porphyria *
Adenosine deaminase deficiency *
Chédiak-Higashi syndrome †
Congenital erythropoietic
  porphyria †
Congenital nephrosis *
Cystinosis *
Familial hypercholesterolemia †
Glutathionuria †
Hypophosphatasia *
I-cell disease *
Leigh's encephalopathy †
Lesch-Nyhan syndrome *

Lysosomal acid phosphatase
  deficiency *
Lysyl-protocollagen hydroxylase
  deficiency †
Myotonic muscular dystrophy †
Nail-Patella syndrome †
Orotic aciduria †
Protoporphyria †
Saccharopinuria †
Sickle cell anemia †
Testicular feminization †
Thalassemia *
Xeroderma pigmentosum *

* prenatal diagnosis possible
† prenatal diagnosis potentially possible

Index